Review for
Therapeutic Massage and Bodywork Certification

Review for

Therapeutic Massage and Bodywork Certification

Joseph Ashton, MS, PT
Duke Cassel, NCTMB

LIPPINCOTT WILLIAMS & WILKINS
A **Wolters Kluwer** Company

Philadelphia • Baltimore • New York • London
Buenos Aires • Hong Kong • Sydney • Tokyo

Acqusitions Editor: Pete Darcy
Managing Editor: Beth Goldner
Marketing Manager: Christen DeMarco
Senior Production Editor: Karen M. Ruppert
Designer: Doug Smock
Compositor: Peirce Graphic Services
Printer: DRC

351 West Camden Street
Baltimore, MD 21201

530 Walnut St.
Philadelphia, PA 19106

Printed in the United States of America

Library of Congress Cataloging-in-Publication Data

Ashton, Joseph.
    Review for therapeutic massage and bodywork certification / Joseph Ashton, Duke Cassel.
        p. cm.
    Includes index.
    ISBN 0-7817-3454-1
        1. Massage therapy.   2. Masseurs—Certification—United States— Study guides.   I. Cassel, Duke.   II. Title.

RM722 .A845 2002
615.8'22'076—dc21

                                                                    2002023562

To purchase additional copies of this book, call our customer service department at **(800) 638-3030** or fax orders to **(301) 824-7390.** International customers should call **(301) 714-2324.**

Visit Lippincott Williams & Wilkins on the Internet: http://www.LWW.com.
Lippincott Williams & Wilkins customer service representatives are available from 8:30 am to 6:00 pm, EST.

                                          02 03 04 05 06
                                    1 2 3 4 5 6 7 8 9 10

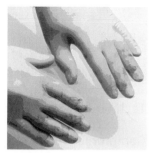

Contents

Preface   *vii*
About the Authors   *ix*

Part I
Human Anatomy, Physiology, and Kinesiology   *1*

1 Introduction: Review of Body Systems   *1*

2 Chemistry Review   *5*

3 Cellular Review   *7*

4 Integumentary System   *11*

5 Skeletal System   *15*

6 Articulations   *25*

7 Muscular System   *31*

8 Nervous System   *49*

9 Sensory System   *55*

10 Endocrine System   *59*

11 Cardiovascular System   *63*

12 Lymphatic and Immune System   *71*

13 Respiratory System   *75*

14 Digestive System   *79*

15 Urinary System   *83*

16 Reproductive System   *87*

17 Craniosacral System   *91*

18 Biomechanics and Kinesiology   *93*

19 Medical Terminology   *97*

20 Oriental Medicine   *101*

21 Other Energy Systems   *105*

Part I Practice Questions   *107*

Part II
Clinical Pathology   *121*

22 History and Client Intake   *121*

23 Introduction to Disease   *125*

24 Diseases of the Integumentary System   *129*

25 Diseases of the Skeletal System   *133*

26 Diseases of the Joints (Articulations)   *135*

27 Diseases of the Muscular
System *139*

28 Diseases of the Nervous
System *141*

29 Diseases of the Sensory
System *145*

30 Diseases of the Endocrine
System *147*

31 Diseases of the Cardiovascular
System *151*

32 Diseases of the Lymphatic and
Immune Systems *155*

33 Diseases of the Respiratory
System *157*

34 Diseases of the Digestive
System *159*

35 Diseases of the Urinary
System *163*

36 Diseases of the Reproductive
System *165*

Part II Practice Questions *169*

Part III
Massage Therapy and
Bodywork: Theory, Assessment,
and Application *175*

37 Introduction to Bodywork *175*

38 Assessment *181*

39 Application: Precautions *185*

40 Application: Positioning *197*

41 Application: Technique *203*

42 Application: Communication *211*

43 Application: Hydrotherapy *213*

44 Application: First Aid
and Cardiopulmonary
Resuscitation *217*

45 Touch Therapy Modalities *227*

46 Holistic Nutrition *235*

47 Holistic Practice *239*

Part III Practice Questions *241*

Part IV
Professional Standards, Ethics,
and Business Practices *253*

48 Ethics *253*

49 Business Practices *255*

Part IV Practice Questions *261*

Part V

Practice Examination *265*
Answer Key *285*

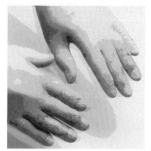

Preface

Review for Therapeutic Massage and Bodywork Certification is a comprehensive review for preparing for the National Certification Examination for Therapeutic Massage and Bodywork. This book provides a simple, easy-to-understand overview of the main concepts and principles for the four main sections of the test:

1. Anatomy, Physiology, and Kinesiology
2. Clinical Pathology
3. Theory of Massage and Bodywork
4. Professional Standards, Ethics, and Business Practices

A full Practice Examination is also included so that you can better prepare yourself to take the exam.

This study guide contains basic definitions and fundamental concepts along with applications of the material and practice questions for each section. Simple diagrams, images, and drawings are included to help the student visualize this material and be able to locate the anatomical structures discussed in each section. I hope you enjoy the simple, basic format and find it easy to study and to reference. I also hope the information and practice questions in this book give you the preparation you need to pass the National Exam.

Good luck on the test!

JOSEPH ASHTON

Review for Therapeutic Massage and Bodywork Certification provides an overview of the information that is fundamental for the serious bodyworker to achieve National Certification standards through the NCTMB. This book covers the main concepts of therapeutic massage as well as concepts necessary for professionalism and business.

This book is not intended to provide exact detail for every condition; therefore, the reader should understand that whenever in doubt about a procedure or condition, contact the client's physician before performing any bodywork.

The advantage to this book is its simplicity and easy-to-understand format. It is also important to note that the text has been compiled by authors who are using this information on a daily basis as teachers in the massage profession. While writing this book, I pulled a great deal from my own experience in preparing for and taking the National Certification Examination.

Finally, this book is also designed to do more than just prepare the potential candidate to pass the National Examination. Unlike other review study guides, this volume also provides additional clinical information to enhance the therapist's ability to perform in a clinical setting.

Good Luck on the Test! Remember, "Massage starts in the Mind".

DUKE E. CASSEL

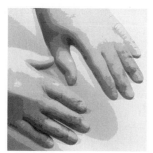

About the Authors

Joseph Ashton earned a Bachelor of Science degree at Brigham Young University and a Master of Science degree at Washington University School of Medicine in St. Louis, Missouri. He began teaching in the Human Anatomy laboratory while still at Brigham Young. Since that time, he has taught Anatomy and Physiology at LDS Business College and Salt Lake Community College in Salt Lake City and at Washington University in St Louis, and he has spent several years teaching and designing the curriculum for the Anatomy and Physiology, Functional Anatomy, General Pathology and Joint Pathology courses at Myotherapy College of Utah. Along with his teaching, he has assisted in writing and editing other anatomical manuals and study guides, including *Human Anatomy and Physiology* from the Schaum's Outline Series published by McGraw-Hill College Publisher.

Duke Cassel is a graduate of the Basic Core Course and the Advanced Therapeutic Bodywork Course at the Myotherapy College of Utah in Salt Lake City, Utah. He has been a licensed massage therapist since 1991 as well as a core instructor at the Myotherapy College of Utah since 1992. He has completed over 1400 hours of training in Spinal Touch, Acutherapy, Hospital Massage, Neuro-link, Reiki I and II, and Craniosacral Therapy. He is Nationally Certified through the National Certification Board for Therapeutic Massage and Bodywork (NCBTMB). Along with teaching, he served as the team sports massage therapist for the Utah Starzz professional women's basketball team. Duke currently practices massage therapy in his own private clinic.

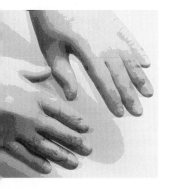

Part I
Human Anatomy, Physiology, and Kinesiology

Chapter One

Introduction: Review of Body Systems

Anatomy — the science of the structure of the body and its parts.
Physiology — the study of the normal functioning of the body.

Body Organization

Cell — the basic unit of life; the basic structural unit that makes up tissue and organs.
Tissue — a group or collection of similar cells that perform a specific function.
Organ — a structure of the body that is made up of a group of tissues and performs a specialized function.
Organ system — a group of organs that act together to perform a specialized body function.
Organism — an individual living thing.

> The human organism starts out as only two cells—a sperm cell and an egg cell (ovum). These two cells continue to multiply and divide as we grow. As mature adults, we have between 60 and 100 trillion cells!

Organ Systems

Integumentary — the skin and the accessory organs in it (e.g., hair, nails, glands) provide external support and protection.
Skeletal — a skeleton of 206 bones and the joints between them provide support and a framework for body movement.
Muscular — the muscles of the body provide movement and body heat.
Nervous — organs such as the brain, spinal cord, and nerves make communication within the body, learning, and memory possible.
Sensory — specialized sense organs (ears, eyes, nose, tongue) make possible the special senses of hearing, sight, smell, and taste.
Circulatory — the heart and blood vessels carry blood to all parts of the body and remove waste products.
Lymphatic — organs such as the spleen, thymus, lymph nodes, and tonsils produce body immunity, drain fluids from tissues, and help absorb fats.
Respiratory — the lungs and air passages bring oxygen into the body and move carbon dioxide out of the body.

Digestive — organs such as the stomach and intestines take in food and break it down into nutrients that the body can use.

Endocrine — internal glands such as the pituitary, thyroid, adrenals, and gonads secrete hormones for body regulation.

Urinary — the kidneys, ureters, bladder, and urethra work together to remove waste products and excess water and transport urine out of the body.

Reproductive — internal and external organs such as the testes, ovaries, penis, vagina, and uterus produce, transport, and provide a proper environment for the gametes or sex cells (i.e., sperm and eggs) to mature and/or unite.

Body Processes

Metabolism — all of the chemical and physical processes that go on inside of the body to sustain life.

> **Catabolism** — the "breaking down" phase of metabolism (i.e., food is broken down into nutrients that the body can use).
>
> **Anabolism** — the "building up" phase of metabolism (i.e., cells take the nutrients that the body has broken down and build their cellular components).

Homeostasis [*homeo = same; stasis = stay*] — a state of balance (or "steady state") that the body maintains to stay alive; maintained through positive and negative feedback systems.

> **Anabolic** steroids are a group of chemicals that promote body growth, particularly growth of muscle tissue. These are the "steroids" that athletes use to increase their strength and performance.

Anatomical Directions

Superior — above; in a higher position.

Inferior — below; in a lower position.

Medial — closer to the midline of the body.

Lateral — farther away from the midline of the body.

Proximal — closer to the main mass of the body.

Distal — farther away from the main mass of the body.

Anterior (ventral) — toward the front surface (i.e., toward the belly).

Posterior (dorsal) — toward the back surface.

Superficial — on the surface.

Deep — lying far down; underneath several layers.

Cephalad — toward the head or cranium.

Caudal [*caud = tail*] — toward the tailbone or sacrum.

> **Anatomical position** is described as standing erect (facing the observer), feet parallel, and arms to the sides with the palms facing forward. It is the reference frame used when studying the body. All of the directions are used to describe the relationship of one body part to another when the body is in anatomical position.

Planes of Division

Frontal plane (coronal plane) — divides the body into anterior and posterior portions.

Sagittal plane — divides the body into right and left portions.

> **Midsagittal plane** — the single plane that divides the body into equal right and left halves.

Transverse plane (horizontal plane) — divides the body into top and bottom portions.

Oblique plane — slanting plane; a plane that is not in any of the other planes.

> Often two terms will be combined to describe a position that is halfway between two other positions (e.g., posterolateral, anteromedial). It is much the same as using terms such as southwest or northeast.

> The frontal, sagittal, and transverse planes are considered the three "cardinal planes."

Body Cavities

Ventral cavity — made up of the thoracic and abdominopelvic cavities.
    Thoracic cavity — the cavity within the rib cage and above the diaphragm; contains the heart, lungs, etc.
        Pericardial cavity — within the thoracic cavity; contains the heart.
    Abdominopelvic cavity — the cavity below the diaphragm; contains the abdominal and pelvic cavities.

> The diaphragm separates the thoracic cavity from the abdominopelvic cavity.

        Abdominal cavity — contains most of the digestive organs, the liver, and the spleen.
    Pelvic cavity — contains the bladder, rectum, and some reproductive organs.
Dorsal cavity — made up of the cranial and spinal cavities.
    Cranial cavity — the cavity within the skull; contains the brain.
    Spinal cavity — the cavity within the spinal column; houses the spinal cord.

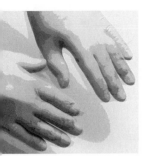

Chapter Two

Chemistry Review

Chemistry Overview

Atom — the smallest unit of any living or nonliving thing (Figure 2–1). The structure of the atom is:

Proton — positively charged particle found in the nucleus of the atom.

Electron — negatively charged particle that orbits the nucleus of the atom.

Neutron — particle with no charge found in the nucleus of the atom.

Element — a substance that consists of atoms with the same chemical properties; classified as atoms with the same number of protons.

Molecule — two or more atoms bonded together; also called a compound.

Macromolecule — a large molecule (e.g., DNA, hemoglobin).

Ion — a positively or negatively charged atom or molecule; an atom or molecule that has had electrons added or taken away.

Electrolyte — a substance that releases ions when put into a solution; electrolytes are necessary for the proper functioning of all cells in the body; some of the more important electrolytes are:

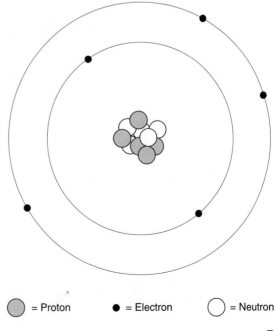

Figure 2–1. This representation of the boron atom illustrates the basic structure of atoms. Note that the element boron contains five neutrons and five protons.

○ = Proton   ● = Electron   ○ = Neutron

5

Sodium (Na$^+$)
Potassium (K$^+$)
Chloride (Cl$^-$)
Magnesium (Mg^{2+})
Calcium (Ca^{2+})
Iodine (I$^-$)

Mixture — a combination of two or more substances.
Solution — a homogeneous mixture of a substance of smaller abundance (solute) dissolved into a substance of greater abundance (solvent).
  Solute — the dissolved substance (e.g., salt, sugar).
  Solvent — the dissolving substance (e.g., water).
Suspension — a mixture of two or more substances in a liquid that do not dissolve but distribute evenly throughout the liquid (e.g., India ink, blood).

Acids and Bases

Common acids include stomach acid (gastric juice), carbonic acid (in carbonated drinks), acetic acid (vinegar), lactic acid, and amino acids. Common bases include sodium bicarbonate (baking soda), ammonia, borax, and bleach.

Acid — a substance that releases hydrogen ions (H$^+$) in a solution; for example, hydrogen chloride (HCl) is an acid because when put in a solution it ionizes into H$^+$ and Cl$^-$ (HCl $\rightarrow$ H$^+$ + Cl$^-$).
Base — a substance that accepts or binds to hydrogen ions (H$^+$) in a solution; for example, sodium hydroxide (NaOH) is a base because in a solution it becomes Na$^+$ and OH$^-$ (NaOH $\rightarrow$ Na$^+$ + OH$^+$), and the OH$^-$ can then bind to any H$^+$ present in the solution.
pH scale — the scale from 0 to 14 used to measure acidity and alkalinity (basicity); a substance with a pH below 7 is considered an acid, while a substance with a pH above 7 is considered a base; the farther the pH is from 7, the stronger the acid or base (Figure 2–2).
Buffer — any substance in a solution that prevents sharp changes in pH.

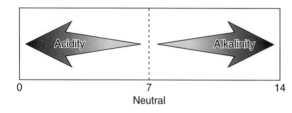

0   7   14
Neutral

Figure 2–2. Diagram illustrating the pH scale.

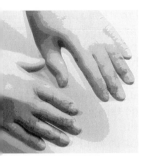

Chapter Three

Cellular Review

Cells

Prokaryote — the term used to describe a cell that does not have a nucleus in which to store its genetic material (e.g., bacteria).

Eukaryote — the term used to describe a cell with an enclosed nucleus in which the cell stores genetic material (e.g., plants, fungi, animals, humans).

Many **antibiotics,** such as penicillin, have been developed to fight bacterial infections. These antibiotics will not destroy the cells of the person who has the infection because the cells are eukaryotic and the bacteria are prokaryotic.

Eukaryotic Cell Structure and Organelles

Cell membrane — the external structure that contains the cell contents and regulates what travels into and out of the cell by way of many different proteins that act as gates, channels, or pumps; composed of a phospholipid bilayer.

Cytoplasm [*cyto = cell; plasma = fluid*] — the fluid that fills the cell; allows the nutrients and building blocks to circulate within the cell.

Nucleus — the largest of the organelles; contains the genetic material, including:

    Deoxyribonucleic acid (DNA) — genetic "master plan" or "blueprint" for the body; contains the genetic information of the cell; assumes the shape of a double helix.

    Chromosomes — thread-like structures made up of DNA; the DNA in the human cell is divided into 23 pairs of chromosomes.

DNA and RNA are composed of only a handful of **nucleotide bases.** The sequence of these bases determines the actual message that is encoded, much like the sequence of letters determines the word that is spelled.

    Genes — segments of chromosomes that carry the genetic code for a specific protein.

    Ribonucleic acid (RNA) — a single-stranded molecule; transfers the genetic information to be translated from the DNA in the nucleus to the cytoplasm of the cell.

Ribosomes — organelles responsible for reading or decoding RNA and using the information to synthesize (assemble) necessary proteins.

Endoplasmic reticulum (ER) — a network of tubules in the cytoplasm responsible for collecting the proteins manufactured by the ribosomes and then packaging and shipping the proteins to different areas of the cell.

    Rough ER — endoplasmic reticulum that has ribosomes bound to its surface; many proteins that are secreted by the cell are produced here.

Smooth ER — endoplasmic reticulum that lacks ribosomes bound to its surface; many enzymes that synthesize important lipids and steroids are contained here.

Golgi apparatus — the center for storing, sorting, modifying, and delivering the products of ribosomes and the endoplasmic reticulum, particularly those products that are to be secreted by the cell (e.g., mucus).

Mitochondria — the organelles responsible for taking energy out of sugars, fats, and other fuels and transferring it to the bonds that hold the adenosine triphosphate molecule together; often referred to as the "powerhouses" of the cell.

Lysosome — a small bag or pocket of digestive enzymes in the cell that is used to digest cells and organelles that are either foreign or damaged.

Centrioles — small, spindle-like organelles that supervise cell division; aid in distributing the DNA evenly into the two daughter cells that result when the parent cell divides.

Cilia — hair-like protrusions from the cell membrane used for moving substances (e.g., mucus, fluids) around the cell.

Flagellum — a tail-like projection on the cell membrane used for cell motility, as on sperm cells.

Mitosis — the process of cell division in which one cell divides into two identical daughter cells.

Tonicity — a measure of the strength of concentration of a solution.

> **Hypertonic** — a solution with a higher concentration of solute.
>
> **Isotonic** — a solution with the same concentration of solute.
>
> **Hypotonic** — a solution with a lower concentration of solute.

The terms hypertonic, isotonic, and hypotonic are used to compare the relative strengths of two solutions. When dealing with cells and body fluids, these terms are used to compare solutions of certain concentrations to "normal" body fluid concentrations.

Transport and Movement of Cells

Diffusion — movement of a substance from an area of high concentration to an area of low concentration in order to reach a uniform concentration.

Osmosis — diffusion of water through a semipermeable membrane.

> **Osmotic pressure** — the pressure created from a solvent, such as water, diffusing across a semipermeable membrane.

Filtration — movement of a fluid through a membrane with pores that restrict larger molecules from passing through but allow the passage of smaller molecules; based on mechanical pressure.

Active transport — transport of substances into or out of the cell that requires energy; transport "uphill" or against a concentration gradient (i.e., from an area of low concentration to an area of high concentration); opposite of diffusion.

Phagocytosis [phago = eat; cyte = cell; sis = process] — the process by which solid particles are engulfed by the cell membrane.

Pinocytosis [pino = drink; cyte = cell; sis = process] — the process by which fluids are engulfed by the cell membrane.

Dialysis — artificial filtering of waste and excess material out of the blood through a semipermeable membrane (see Chapter 35 for a detailed description of hemodialysis and peritoneal dialysis).

Tissues

Histology — the study of tissues.

Epithelial tissue — tissue that lines body surfaces and cavities.

Squamous epithelial tissue [*squamous = flat*] — composed of flattened cells; well adapted for diffusion, filtration, and protection; found in the skin, the interior of blood vessels, the alveoli of the lungs, and the glomerulus in the kidney.

Cuboidal epithelial tissue — composed of cube-shaped cells; found lining secretory, excretory, and absorptive glands and ducts (e.g., sweat glands, salivary glands, kidney tubules).

Columnar epithelial tissue — column-shaped cells used for protection and, in some cases, production of mucus; found in the linings of the digestive and respiratory systems and in the uterine tubes; some types possess cilia.

Transitional epithelial tissue — similar to squamous epithelium in shape; adapted for distension (stretching); found in the urinary tract only, particularly in the bladder.

Connective tissue — tissue used for packaging, protecting, and supporting various organs; most abundant tissue in the body; found in almost every region and organ of the body.

Soft connective tissue includes:

Adipose tissue [*adiposus = fat*] — made up of adipose cells that store fat molecules; helps insulate the body and store energy.

Fascia — the lining around muscles, blood vessels, and nerves that connects them to the surrounding tissues to hold them in place.

Dense fibrous connective tissue — strong but flexible tissue used to bind muscle to bone or bone to bone; found in tendons, ligaments, scars, and the renal capsule (see Chapter 15).

> Ligaments and tendons that are damaged may take a long time to heal primarily because they have poor blood supply.

  Tendon — tissue that connects muscle to bone or other tissue.

  Ligament [*ligare = bind*] — tissue that connects bone to bone.

Reticular connective tissue — tissue woven from a network of fibers with some phagocytes (i.e., cells that engulf and destroy foreign or damaged cells); found in the spleen, blood vessels, lymph nodes, and bone marrow.

Hard connective tissue includes:

Bone — the most rigid connective tissue; provides structure and protection.

Cartilage (gristle) — a semisolid, somewhat elastic connective tissue; found in the ears, nose, and joints.

Liquid connective tissue includes:

Blood (hematopoietic tissue) — specialized cells (erythrocytes, leukocytes, thrombocytes) suspended in the liquid plasma.

Muscle tissue — tissue responsible for body movement and movement in the body.

Smooth muscle tissue (visceral muscle tissue) — muscle tissue found in the hollow organs of the body (e.g., digestive tract, arterial walls, respiratory passages); responsible for movement in the body; under involuntary control; nonstriated.

Cardiac muscle tissue — muscle tissue found in the heart; produces regular contractions to pump blood through the heart; under involuntary control; striated; cells contain intercalated discs.

  Intercalated discs — small discs at the end of each cell that connect the cells together and allow the spread of an electrical activation from one cell to the cells around it.

Skeletal muscle tissue — muscle tissue attached to the skeleton; responsible for locomotion; under voluntary control; striated.

Nervous tissue — tissue responsible for conducting an action potential (nerve impulse) through the body, allowing tissues to communicate.

Neuron — nerve cell responsible for conducting the action potential; basic unit of the nervous system.

Myelin — made up of neuroglial cells that wrap around neurons to provide support and protection.

Membranes

Mucous membranes (mucosa) — secrete mucus, a thick fluid-like substance; line most of the cavities in the respiratory and digestive systems to protect and lubricate.

Serous membranes (serosa) — secrete serous fluid, a lubricant; cover the internal organs in the thoracic, abdominal, and pelvic cavities.

Pleurae — serous membranes associated with the lungs.

Pericardium — serous membrane surrounding the heart.

Peritoneum — serous membrane of the abdominopelvic cavity.

Synovial membranes — the highly vascular membranes that surround the inside of joint capsules in synovial joints (i.e., freely moveable joints); secrete synovial fluid (also called synovium), a lubricant, into the joint cavity.

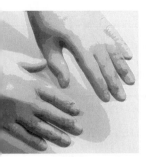

Chapter Four

Integumentary System

〽 Layers of the Integument (Figure 4–1)

Epidermis — superficial layer; composed mostly of squamous epithelial cells.
    Stratum corneum — outermost layer of the skin; cells produced in the stratum basale are pushed up into the stratum corneum by newer cells being produced; the last few layers of the stratum corneum are dead cells that are continually shed.
        Keratin — a protein found in the stratum corneum that makes this layer tough and impenetrable.

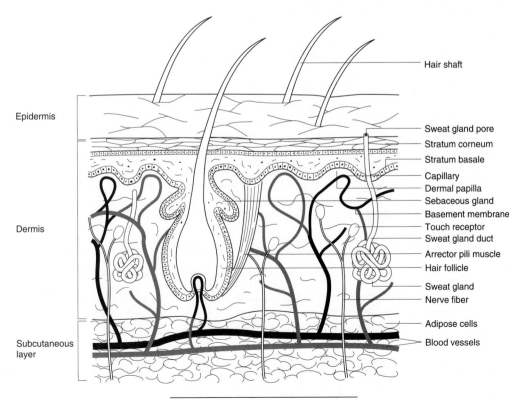

Figure 4–1. Layers of the integument.

Stratum basale — innermost layer of the epidermis; cells in this layer are constantly dividing and pushing the layers upward toward the stratum corneum (the cells die as they move away from the nutrient and oxygen supply found in this layer).

> In approximately 6 to 8 weeks, skin cells move from the stratum basale to the stratum corneum, where they are shed.

> **Melanin** — a dark pigment in the skin and hair that is produced by melanocytes found in the stratum basale; protects against the ultraviolet rays of the sun.

Dermis — the layer below the epidermis of the skin; composed of connective tissues, blood vessels, glands, muscle tissue, nerve endings, and hair follicles.

> Because all races have the same number of melanocytes, skin color is determined by the amount of melanin produced. An **albino** has a genetic disorder in which the melanocytes cannot produce melanin, leaving the skin characteristically white or without color.

> **Arrector pili** — the muscle attached to the root of the hair; contracts when the person is scared or when the skin becomes chilled to produce body heat; responsible for creating "goose bumps."

> **Blood vessels** — bring blood to the epidermis and regulate body temperature; when body temperature rises, these blood vessels fill with blood, bringing the heat closer to the surface of the skin and allowing it to dissipate by evaporating sweat.

> **Nerve endings** — general sensory receptors for pressure, temperature, and pain.

Subcutaneous layer (superficial fascia, hypodermis) — the last layer of the integument; composed mostly of connective tissues (primarily adipose tissue) and blood vessels; varies in thickness depending on its location in the body and on the age, sex, and overall health of the individual.

Appendages to the Integument

Sebaceous glands — glands located along the shaft of the hair; secrete sebum, an oily substance, along the shaft of the hair that disperses along the surface of the skin and keeps the stratum corneum supple and waterproof.

Sudoriferous glands [*sudorifer = sweat*] — glands that produce and secrete perspiration (sweat), a fluid that is approximately 99% water and contains some electrolytes, salts, and urea; sweat eliminates some wastes and cools the body by removing heat through evaporation.

> **Eccrine glands** — most numerous type of sweat gland; found throughout the body, particularly on the back, forehead, hands, and feet.

> **Apocrine glands** — larger sweat glands located in the axillary and pubic regions; secrete a more viscous and odoriferous secretion; become active at puberty.

> **Mammary glands** — specialized sudoriferous glands in the breasts that secrete milk.

Ceruminous glands [*cera = wax*] — specialized secretory glands located in the external ear canal that secrete cerumen (earwax).

Hair — consists of a shaft, root, and bulb; provides limited protection (e.g., eyelashes protect the eye, hair in the nostrils protects the nose).

> The shaft of the hair is made up of dead, keratinized tissue that develops from the **bulb** in the **hair follicle**. Hair grows approximately 1 mm every 3 days, and a healthy person may lose up to 100 hairs in 1 day.

Fingernails and toenails — hardened layer of the stratum corneum found at the end of each finger and toe; helps protect the end of the digits and aids in picking up objects with the fingers.

Functions of the Integumentary System

Protection — protects against dehydration and invasion of pathogenic organisms.

Temperature regulation — produces and secretes sweat; diverts blood to the superficial layers of the skin to dissipate heat.

Sensory reception — receptors in the skin respond to pain, touch, pressure, and temperature.

Cutaneous absorption — skin absorbs ultraviolet light and some oxygen and carbon dioxide.

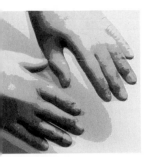

Chapter Five

Skeletal System

Bone Tissue (Osseous Tissue)

Osteocytes [*osteo = bone; cyte = cell*] — individual bone cells.
    Osteoclasts [*clast = break*] — bone cells that produce substances that break down bone tissue to remove unneeded tissue and, more importantly, release stored minerals like calcium and phosphate.
    Osteoblasts [*blast = generative*] — bone cells that build up or repair bone tissue, thus storing important minerals for future use.

Bone Shapes

Long bones — bones that are longer than they are wide; act as levers; examples include the humerus, radius, ulna, femur, tibia, fibula, metacarpus, and phalanges.
Short bones — square or cube-shaped bones; examples include the carpus and tarsus.
Flat bones — bones with broad surfaces for muscle attachment; examples include the cranial bones, scapula, ribs, and ilium.
Irregular bones — bones with varied shapes; examples include the vertebrae and some facial and cranial bones.

Bone Structure

Diaphysis — the shaft of a long bone.
Epiphyses — the ends of a long bone.
    Epiphyseal plate — the "growth plate;" the area of the epiphysis where mitotic division of bone cells takes place, allowing the shaft to increase in length.
Articular cartilage — a layer of hyaline cartilage that lines the surfaces of bones where they connect to other bones.
Medullary cavity — the cavity in the diaphysis of long bones.
Periosteum — a layer of tissue that covers the surfaces of bones; provides a connective layer around the bone to which tendons can attach.
    Sharpey's fibers — small fibers that connect the periosteum to the surface of the bone.
Compact bone — the dense outer layer of bone; makes up the shafts of long bones and the outer layer of other bones.

Shin splints is a common disorder experienced by athletes. It is brought on by sudden overuse of the muscles of the anterior or posterior calf. This trauma to the muscles and their attachment at the periosteum produces inflammation and pain around the shins.

Spongy bone — bone tissue that contains many porous spaces, causing it to look "spongy"; found in the epiphyses of long bones and in the interior of other bones.

Bone marrow — the soft material made up of a meshwork of connective tissue that is found in the cavities of bones.

> **Red marrow** — tissue found mostly in the spongy bone that produces the blood cells.
>
> **Yellow marrow** — fatty tissue found in the medullary cavity.

Functions of Bones

1. Serve as a framework for the body
2. Protect delicate organs such as the brain, spinal cord, lungs, and eyes
3. Serve as levers for the muscles to act upon to produce body movement
4. Serve as a storehouse for minerals such as calcium and phosphorus
5. Produce red blood cells, white blood cells, and platelets (in the marrow)

The Skeleton

Terminology

Processes — "bumps" found on the surfaces of bones.
> **Tubercle** — a small, rounded bump used for muscle attachment.
> **Tuberosity** — a large, roughened bump.
> **Spine** — a sharp, pointed bump.
> **Condyle** — a rounded bump for bone articulation.
> **Epicondyle** — a bump above a condyle.
> **Crest** — a ridge.
> **Line** — a long bump.

Depressions and openings — hollow or depressed areas; an orifice or open space.
> **Foramen** — a rounded hole through a bone (plural is foramina).
> **Fossa** — a shallow depression in a bone.
> **Groove** — a long depression; a furrow in a bone.
> **Sinus** — a cavity in a bone.
> **Meatus** — a canal in a bone.
> **Fissure** — a long, narrow depression.

Suture — where two bones in the skull have grown together and joined.

The following is a list of the bones in the axial and appendicular skeletons and their main features (e.g., processes, foramina). Particular care was taken to include the processes that will be discussed in Chapter 6 as parts of bones that make up the joints and in Chapter 7 as origins or insertions for particular muscles. Practice finding and identifying each bone and its landmarks on the diagrams and on your own body so that you will be able to recognize each bone when studying muscle origins and insertions.

Axial Skeleton

Skull *(Figure 5–1)*
Frontal bone
Parietal bones
Temporal bones
  External auditory meatus
  Mastoid process
  Styloid process
Nasal bones
Lacrimal bones
Zygomatic bone
  Zygomatic arch
Maxillary bone (maxilla)
  Palatine process
Occipital bone
  Occipital condyles
  Foramen magnum
Sphenoid bone
  Sella turcica
  Pterygoid plates

Sutures
Coronal suture
Sagittal suture
Lambdoid suture
Squamous suture

Head and Neck
Mandible
  Condyloid process
  Coronoid process
  Ramus
  Angle of the mandible
Hyoid bone
Ear ossicles
  Malleus
  Incus
  Stapes

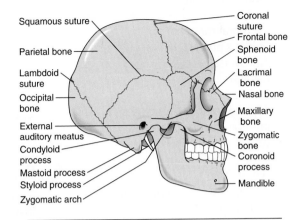

Figure 5–1. Diagram of the skull—right lateral view.

Vertebral Column *(Figure 5–2)*

Vertebrae (terminology)
- Body
- Vertebral foramen
- Spinous process
- Transverse process
- Lamina
- Pedicle
- Superior articular processes
- Inferior articular processes

Cervical vertebrae (7)
- Atlas (C1)
- Axis (C2)
  - Dens (odontoid process)
- Transverse foramen

Thoracic vertebrae (12)
- Articular facets

Lumbar vertebrae (5)

Sacral vertebrae

Coccyx ("tailbone")

Thorax

Ribs (12 pairs total)
- True ribs (7 pairs)
- False ribs (3 pairs)
- Floating ribs (2 pairs)

Sternum *(Figure 5–3)*

- Clavicular notch
- Manubrium
- Body
- Xiphoid process

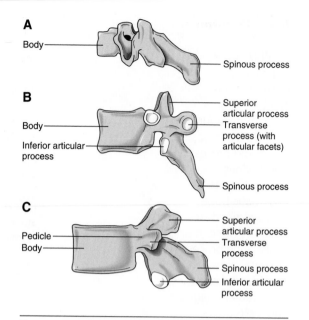

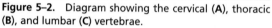

Figure 5–2. Diagram showing the cervical (**A**), thoracic (**B**), and lumbar (**C**) vertebrae.

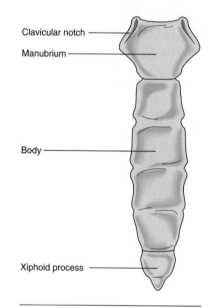

Figure 5–3. Diagram of the sternum—anterior view.

Appendicular Skeleton—Upper Extremities

Shoulder Girdle

Clavicle ("collar bone")
- Sternal end
- Acromial end

Scapula ("shoulder blade") [*Figure 5–4*]
Medial (vertebral) border
Lateral (axillary) border
Spine of scapula
Acromion process
Coracoid process
Supraspinous fossa
Infraspinous fossa
Subscapular fossa
Glenoid fossa

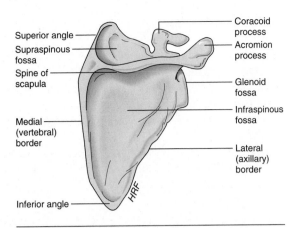

Figure 5–4. Diagram of the right scapula—posterior view.

Arms and Hands
Humerus *(Figure 5–5)*
Greater tubercle
Lesser tubercle
Bicipital groove
Deltoid tuberosity
Medial epicondyle
Lateral epicondyle
Trochlea
Capitulum

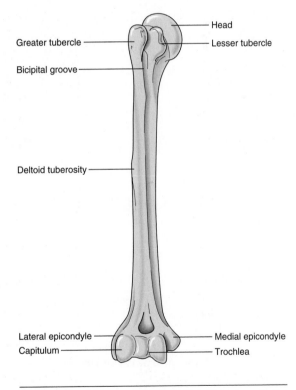

Figure 5–5. Diagram of the right humerus—anterior view.

Radius *(Figure 5–6)*
    Head
    Radial tuberosity
    Styloid process

Ulna *(see Figure 5–6)*
    Ulnar tuberosity
    Olecranon process
    Coronoid process
    Styloid process

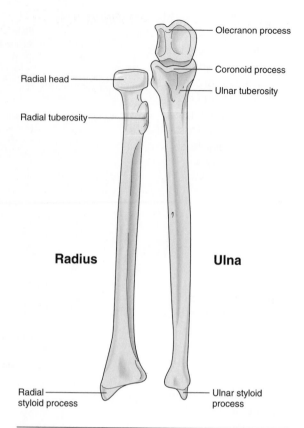

Figure 5–6. Diagram of the right radius and ulna—anterior view.

Carpus (8 carpals per hand) [*Figure 5–7*]
    Scaphoid bone
    Lunate bone
    Triquetral bone
    Pisiform bone
    Trapezium bone
    Trapezoid bone
    Capitate bone
    Hamate bone

Metacarpus (5 metacarpals per hand)
    [*see Figure 5–7*]
    I through V

Phalanges (14 per hand) [*see Figure 5–7*]
    Proximal phalanges
    Middle phalanges
    Distal phalanges

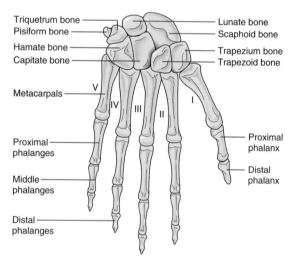

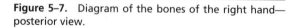

Figure 5–7. Diagram of the bones of the right hand—posterior view.

Appendicular Skeleton—Lower Extremities

Pelvic Girdle *(Figure 5–8)*

Os coxae
  Ilium
    Iliac crest
    Iliac fossa
    Greater sciatic notch
    Iliac spines
      Anterior superior iliac spine (ASIS)
      Anterior inferior iliac spine (AIIS)
      Posterior superior iliac spine (PSIS)
      Posterior inferior iliac spine (PIIS)
  Ischium
    Ischial tuberosity
    Ramus
    Ischial spine
  Pubis
    Pubic crest
    Superior ramus
    Inferior ramus
    Pubic symphysis
Obturator foramen
Acetabulum

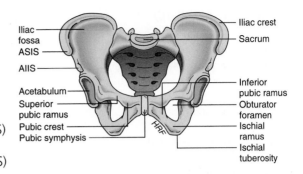

Figure 5–8. Diagram of the pelvis—anterior view. *AIIS* = anterior inferior iliac spine; *ASIS* = anterior superior iliac spine.

Legs and Feet
Femur *(Figure 5–9)*

  Head
  Neck
  Greater trochanter
  Lesser trochanter
  Intertrochanteric crest
  Gluteal tuberosity
  Linea aspera
  Medial condyle
  Lateral condyle
  Medial epicondyle
  Lateral epicondyle
  Intercondylar notch
  Patellar surface

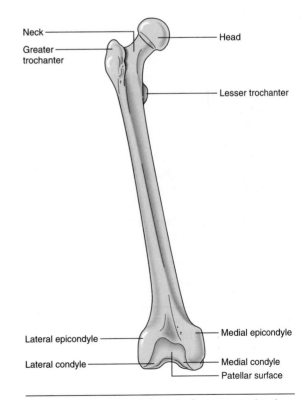

Figure 5–9. Diagram of the right femur—anterior view.

Patella *(Figure 5–10)*

Tibia *(see Figure 5–10)*
  Medial condyle
  Lateral condyle
  Intercondylar eminence
  Tibial tuberosity
  Anterior crest
  Medial malleolus

Fibula *(see Figure 5–10)*
  Head
  Lateral malleolus

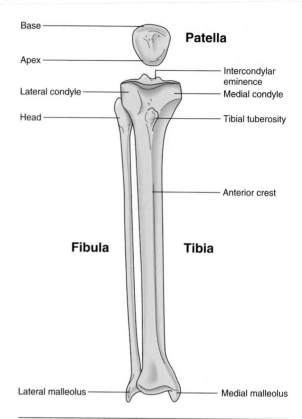

Figure 5–10. Diagram of the right patella, tibia, and fibula—anterior view.

Tarsus (7 tarsals per foot) *[Figure 5–11]*
  Calcaneal bone
  Talus bone
  Navicular bone
  Cuboid bone
  First cuneiform bone
  Second cuneiform bone
  Third cuneiform bone

Metatarsus (5 metatarsals per foot)
  [see Figure 5–11]
  I through V

Phalanges (14 per foot)
  [see Figure 5–11]
  Proximal phalanges
  Middle phalanges
  Distal phalanges

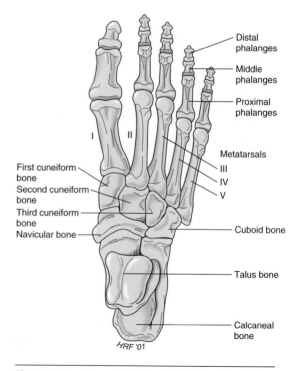

Figure 5–11. Diagram of the right foot—dorsal view.

BIBLIOGRAPHY

Moore KL: *Clinically Oriented Anatomy,* 3rd ed. Baltimore, Williams & Wilkins, 1992, p 444.
Van De Graaf KM: *Human Anatomy,* 4th ed. Dubuque, Wm. C. Brown, 1995, p 325.

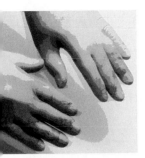

Chapter Six

Articulations

Classification of Joints

Fibrous joints — immovable joints; also called synarthrodial joints; examples include sutures and epiphyseal (growth) plates.

Cartilaginous joints — slightly movable joints; articulating surfaces of the bones are separated by a piece of cartilage; also called amphiarthroses; examples include the intervertebral disks and the pubic symphysis.

Synovial joints — freely movable joints; possess a joint cavity encapsulated by ligamentous structures (joint capsule and/or ligaments); contain synovial fluid that is secreted by the synovial membrane; ends of joints are lined with **hyaline cartilage;** also called diarthroses.

Six types of synovial joints:

Hinge joints — joints that act just like a door on hinges; permit movement in only one plane; examples include the elbow, knee, and interphalangeal joints.

Condylar (ellipsoidal) joints — joints formed by a convex surface within a concave surface; permit movement in two planes; examples include the radiocarpal (wrist) and metacarpophalangeal (base of the fingers) joints.

Gliding (plane) joints — joints formed by two flat surfaces coming together; allow side-to-side movement, back-and-forth movement, and rotation; examples include the intercarpal and intertarsal joints and the facet joints in the spine.

Saddle joints — joints formed by two saddle-shaped surfaces (convex in one plane, concave in another plane); allow for stabilized movement in two planes; an example is the carpometacarpal joint in the thumb.

Ball-and-socket joints — joints formed by a round, convex surface in a socket or cavity; allow movement in all planes (joint with most movement); examples include the glenohumeral (shoulder) and hip joints.

Pivot joints — joints formed by a cone-shaped surface of one bone articulating with a concave notch of another bone; allow rotation only; examples include the atlantoaxial (between C1 and C2) and radioulnar joints.

Joint Movements

Flexion — a bending movement; decreasing the angle between the anterior surfaces of the bones (except at the knees and toes); examples include bending the elbow, bending the knee, making a fist, bending at the waist to pick something up, pulling the leg up at the hip to step up a stair, bowing your head.

Extension — a straightening movement; increasing the angle between bones to 180°; a return from flexion (i.e., a movement opposite of flexion).

Hyperextension — increasing the angle between bones past 180°; for example, looking up at the sky hyperextends the neck.

Abduction — movement away from the midline of the body; examples include bringing the arms upward on the side of the body and opening the legs during a jumping jack (abducts the shoulder and the hip) and spreading the fingers apart.

Adduction — movement toward the midline of the body; examples include bringing the arms downward on the side of the body during a jumping jack and bringing the fingers together from a spread position.

> The terms **ulnar deviation** (adduction) and **radial deviation** (abduction) are often used to describe **wrist** movements. These terms define in which direction the wrist is moving regardless of the position of the subject.

Supination — rolling the forearm so that the palm faces anteriorly (when in anatomical position).

Pronation — rolling the forearm so that the palm faces posteriorly (when in anatomical position).

Rotation — movement around the long axis of the bone.

  External (lateral) rotation — rotating the anterior segment of the bone laterally.

  Internal (medial) rotation — rotating the anterior segment of the bone medially.

  Right and left rotation — rotation of the trunk or neck to the right or left.

> Clapping your hands with your arms at your sides and your elbows bent to 90° uses both external and internal rotation of the shoulder.

Circumduction — a circular or cone-shaped movement involving a combination of flexion, extension, abduction, and adduction; for example, drawing a circle on a chalkboard with a straight elbow.

Elevation — lifting a body part upward; examples include shrugging the shoulders and closing the mouth.

Depression — moving a body part downward; examples include opening the mouth and pulling the shoulders down from a shrugged position.

Dorsiflexion — pulling the top or dorsal surface of the foot up; for example, pulling the toes off of the ground when standing.

Plantar flexion — pointing the plantar surface of the foot downward; for example, standing on the tips of the toes.

Eversion — rolling the sole of the foot to face more laterally; for example, standing on the inside of the foot.

Inversion — rolling the sole of the foot to face more medially; for example, standing on the outside of the foot.

Protraction — moving a body part forward; examples include pushing the jaw forward, bringing the head forward, and pulling the scapulae forward as in a forward reach.

Retraction — moving a body part backward; examples include pulling the jaw in after being pushed out and moving the scapulae toward the spine as in a rowing motion.

Horizontal abduction — moving an abducted body part backward in the transverse or horizontal plane; examples include drawing the string of a bow back and lowering the body down in a push-up.

Horizontal adduction — moving an abducted body part forward in the transverse or horizontal plane; examples include throwing a discus and pushing the body up in a push-up.

Lateral flexion — bending the trunk or neck laterally; also called side bending.

Joints of the Body

Table 6–1 lists the joints with their joint types and the bones that comprise them.

Table 6–1. *The Joints of the Body*

Joint	Joint Type	Bones that Comprise the Joint
Atlanto-occipital	Condylar	Occipital condyles on C1 (atlas)
Atlantoaxial	Pivot	C1 on C2 (atlas on axis)
Intervertebral	Cartilaginous	Vertebral bodies
Temporomandibular (TMJ)	Modified hinge	Condyloid process of the mandible in the mandibular fossa of the temporal bone
Scapulothoracic	Gliding (but not considered a synovial joint)	Scapula on the rib cage
Sternoclavicular	Gliding	Clavicle and manubrium of the sternum
Acromioclavicular (AC)	Gliding	Acromion process and lateral clavicle
Glenohumeral (shoulder)	Ball-and-socket	Head of the humerus in the glenoid fossa
Humeroulnar (elbow)	Hinge	Distal humerus, head of the radius, and semilunar notch of the ulna
Radioulnar	Pivot	Between the radius and ulna, distal and proximal ends
Radiocarpal (wrist)	Condylar	Distal radius and proximal row of the carpus
Intercarpal	Gliding	Adjacent carpal bones
Carpometacarpal	Unspecified	Distal row of carpal and metacarpal bones
Metacarpophalangeal (MCP)	Condylar	Metacarpals and proximal phalanges
Interphalangeal (fingers and toes)		
Proximal interphalangeal (PIP)	Hinge	Proximal phalanges and middle phalanges
Distal interphalangeal (DIP)	Hinge	Middle phalanges and distal phalanges
Sacroiliac (SI)	Gliding	Sacrum and posterior ilium
Hip	Ball-and-socket	Head of the femur in the acetabulum
Tibiofemoral (knee)	Hinge	Distal femur and proximal tibia
Talocrural (ankle)	Hinge	Tibia, fibula, and talus
Subtalar	Hinge	Talus and calcaneus
Midtarsal	Gliding	Talus, calcaneus, navicular, and cuboid

(continued)

Table 6–1. *The Joints of the Body (Continued)*

Joint	Joint Type	Bones that Comprise the Joint
Intertarsal	Gliding	Other adjacent tarsal bones
Tarsometatarsal	Unspecified	Distal row of tarsal and metatarsal bones
Metatarsophalangeal (MTP)	Condylar	Metatarsals and proximal phalanges

Movements and Ranges of Motion for the Major Joints of the Body (Table 6–2)

Table 6–2. *Movements and Ranges for the Major Joints of the Body*

Joint	Joint Type	Movements	Range of Motion (ROM)
Sternoclavicular	Gliding	Protraction	30°
		Retraction	20°
		Elevation	60°
		Depression	20°
Glenohumeral (shoulder)	Ball-and-socket	Flexion	180°
		Extension	50°
		Abduction	180°
		Hyperadduction	50°
		External rotation	90°
		Internal rotation	90°
Humeroulnar (elbow)	Hinge	Flexion	140°
Radioulnar	Pivot	Supination	80°
		Pronation	80°
Radiocarpal (wrist)	Condylar	Flexion	60°
		Extension	60°
		Radial deviation	30°
		Ulnar deviation	20°
Intercarpal	Gliding	Slight gliding movements	N/A
Metacarpo-phalangeal	Condylar	Flexion	90°
		Extension	5°–10°
		Abduction	20°
Intervertebral Cervical	Cartilaginous	Flexion	40°
		Extension	75°
		Lateral flexion	35°
		Rotation	50°
Thoracic	Cartilaginous	Flexion	55°
		Extension	25°
		Lateral flexion	20°
		Rotation	35°

(continued)

Table 6–2. *Movements and Ranges for the Major Joints of the Body (Continued)*

Joint	Joint Type	Movements	Range of Motion (ROM)
Lumbar	Cartilaginous	Flexion	60°
		Extension	35°
		Lateral flexion	20°
		Rotation	5°
Hip	Ball-and-socket	Flexion	100°
		Extension	30°
		Abduction	40°
		Adduction	20°
		External rotation	50°
		Internal rotation	40°
Tibiofemoral (knee)	Hinge	Flexion	135°–145°
Talocrural (ankle)	Hinge	Plantarflexion	40°
		Dorsiflexion	20°
Subtalar	Hinge	Eversion	20°
		Inversion	40°

Major Ligaments of the Body

Nuchal ligament — binds spinous processes of the cervical vertebrae together; serves as the origin for the trapezius and splenius capitis muscles.

Acromioclavicular (AC) ligament — binds the distal end of the clavicle with the acromion process; injured in a shoulder separation.

Transverse carpal ligament (flexor retinaculum) — covers the tendons for the wrist and finger flexors; forms the **carpal tunnel.**

Anterior cruciate ligament (ACL) — connects the femur to the tibia; commonly damaged in athletic knee injuries.

Medial collateral ligament (MCL) — connects the tibia and the femur on the medial aspect of the knee joint; commonly injured in athletic knee injuries.

Anterior talofibular ligament — binds the distal fibula with the talus; crosses the anterolateral aspect of the ankle joint; one of the ligaments most often sprained; usually damaged in a common ankle sprain.

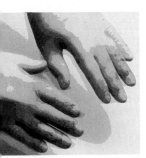

Chapter Seven

Muscular System

Skeletal Muscle Tissue

Functions of Muscle Tissue

1. Body movement
2. Heat production
3. Posture and support

Arrangement of Muscle Tissue

Actin — small, round proteins that form the backbone of the thin myofilaments.

Myosin — long proteins with globular heads; responsible for binding with the actin molecules and pulling the thin myofilaments closer together.

Motor unit — one motor neuron and the many muscle fibers it innervates.

> The arrangement of muscle tissue from the largest to the smallest structure is as follows: **muscle → fasciculus (bundle of muscle fibers) → muscle fiber (muscle cell) → myofibril → thick and thin myofilament → actin and myosin** proteins.

Muscle Contraction

The strength of a muscle contraction is determined by recruitment and the all-or-none law.

Recruitment — the number of motor units activated to perform a given task.

All-or-none law — when a muscle fiber is stimulated by an action potential from a nerve, the entire muscle fiber contracts; motor units also follow this law (when a motor unit is activated, all of the muscle fibers in that unit contract).

Muscle twitch — a single muscle contraction followed by relaxation of the muscle.

Tetanus — a sustained muscle contraction; also called "muscle spasm."

Isometric contraction [*iso = same; metric = length*] — the muscle contracts but does not change length during the contraction.

> Every muscle fiber (muscle cell) belongs to a **motor unit** and therefore receives a branch from an axon terminal. Large muscle groups, such as those in the back or legs concerned with gross motor movements, contain large motor units (approximately 200 to 500 muscle fibers per motor unit). Small muscle groups, such as those around the eyes or in the hands concerned with fine motor movements, are quite small (sometimes only 10 to 25 muscle fibers per motor unit).

Isotonic contraction [*iso = same; tonic = strength or tone*] — the muscle contracts and changes length during the contraction.

Concentric contraction — the muscle contracts and shortens.

Eccentric contraction — the muscle contracts and lengthens.

> **Isometric** contractions stabilize a body part to keep it from moving during an activity. **Concentric** contractions accelerate a body part to produce a force. **Eccentric** contractions slow a body part down or resist a force after it has been produced.

Muscle Movement

Agonist (prime mover) — the muscle that is most responsible for a particular movement when that muscle contracts.

Synergist — a muscle that helps another muscle (an "agonist") perform a movement.

Antagonist — a muscle that works against the agonist or performs the opposite movement.

Muscle Attachment

Tendon — dense, fibrous connective tissue that connects muscle to bone (a **ligament** is connective tissue that connects bone to bone).

Aponeurosis — a broad, flat, thin tendon.

Origin — the more stationary attachment site.

Insertion — the more moveable attachment site.

The Skeletal Muscles of the Body

The main muscles of the body are discussed next. The position, origin, insertion, and action are included for each muscle. The muscles of each anatomical region are grouped into functional groups to show how certain muscles work together to produce joint movements. Use the diagrams to find the positions of the muscles and then practice finding them on your own body.

Muscles of the Face and Head (Figure 7–1; Table 7–1)

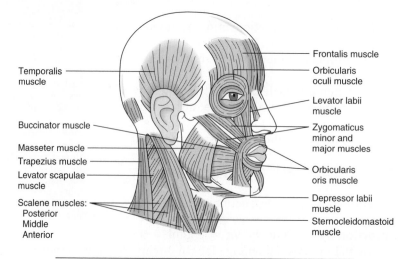

Figure 7–1. Lateral view of the muscles of the face and neck.

Table 7–1. *Muscles of the Face and Head*

Muscle	Position	Origin	Insertion	Action
Frontalis	Forehead	Frontal bone	Eyebrow	Wrinkles forehead; raises eyebrow
Orbicularis oculi	Surrounds the eyes (superficial)	Bones medial to the eye	Eyelid	Closes eyes
Orbicularis oris	Surrounds the mouth (superficial)	Fascia surrounding the mouth	Lips	Closes and purses (puckers) lips
Buccinator	Deep cheek	Maxilla and mandible	Orbicularis oris on corner of mouth	Brings cheeks close to teeth
Zygomaticus muscles	Upper cheek (superficial)	Zygomatic bone	Tissue in the corners of the mouth	Elevates the corners of the mouth ("smiling" muscle)
Levator labii superioris	Above the upper lip, lateral to the nose	Maxilla and zygomatic bone	Upper lip	Elevates upper lip
Depressor labii inferioris	Below the lower lip	Mandible	Lower lip	Depresses lower lip
Masseter	Posterior region of the cheeks (superficial)	Zygomatic arch	Ramus of mandible	Elevates mandible, moves jaw laterally
Temporalis	Lateral cranium (mostly over temporal bone)	Temporal fossa	Coronoid process of mandible	Elevates mandible, retracts mandible
Medial pterygoid	Behind ramus of mandible	Pterygoid plate (medial surface)	Medial ramus of mandible	Elevates jaw, protracts jaw, moves jaw laterally
Lateral pterygoid	Behind ramus of mandible	Pterygoid plate (lateral surface)	Inferior to condyloid process of mandible	Protracts jaw, moves jaw laterally

The masseter, temporalis, medial pterygoid, and lateral pterygoid muscles are the **muscles of mastication** (chewing). The other muscles are used for expression or control of food in the mouth.

Muscles of the Neck (Figure 7–2; Table 7–2; see Figure 7–1)

Flexors:
    Sternocleidomastoid muscle
    Scalene muscles
    Platysma muscle
Extensors:
    Splenius capitis muscle
    Trapezius muscle (upper portion)
Lateral flexors:
    Sternocleidomastoid muscle
    Scalene muscles
    Splenius capitis muscle
Rotators:
    Sternocleidomastoid muscle
    Splenius capitis muscle

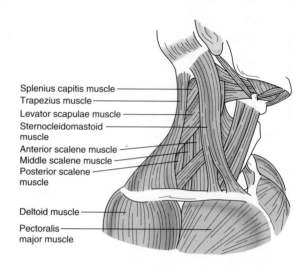

Splenius capitis muscle
Trapezius muscle
Levator scapulae muscle
Sternocleidomastoid muscle
Anterior scalene muscle
Middle scalene muscle
Posterior scalene muscle

Deltoid muscle
Pectoralis major muscle

Figure 7–2. Lateral view of the muscles of the neck.

Muscles That Act on the Scapula (Table 7–3)

Elevators:
    Trapezius muscle (upper portion)
    Levator scapulae muscle

Table 7–2. *Muscles of the Neck*

Muscle	Position	Origin	Insertion	Action
Sternocleido-mastoid	Crosses over the neck from lateral to anterior	Manubrium of sternum; clavicle	Mastoid process of temporal bone	Bilaterally: neck flexion Unilaterally: lateral flexion, neck rotation
Platysma	Covers anterior neck from the mandible to the clavicle	Fascia covering clavicles, sternum, and lower neck	Inferior border of mandible	Depresses lower lip and jaw, neck flexion
Scalenes (anterior, middle, posterior)	Lateral side of the neck	Transverse processes of cervical vertebrae	Anterior: 1st rib Middle: 1st rib Posterior: 2nd rib	Bilaterally: raise first two ribs, assist in neck flexion Unilaterally: lateral flexion of neck
Splenius capitis	Posterior aspect of the neck below the occiput region	Nuchal ligament and spinous processes of C7–T3	Occipital bone and mastoid process	Bilaterally: neck extension Unilaterally: neck rotation, lateral flexion

Protractors:
　　Pectoralis minor muscle
　　Serratus anterior muscle
Upward rotators:
　　Trapezius muscle (upper portion)
　　Trapezius muscle (lower portion)
　　Serratus anterior muscle
Depressors:
　　Trapezius muscle (lower portion)
　　Pectoralis minor muscle
Retractors:
　　Trapezius muscle (middle portion)
　　Rhomboid muscles
Downward rotators:
　　Levator scapulae muscle
　　Rhomboid muscles
　　Pectoralis minor muscle

Table 7–3. *Muscles that Act on the Scapula*

Muscle	Position	Origin	Insertion	Action
Trapezius (upper, middle, and lower portions)	Upper back (superficial)	Occiput, nuchal ligament, and spinous processes of C7–T12	Upper: lateral clavicle and acromion process Middle: spine of scapula Lower: root of the spine of the scapula	Upper: elevation, upward rotation Middle: retraction Lower: depression, upward rotation
Levator scapulae	Under the trapezius, on the lateral side of the neck	Spinous processes of C1–C4	Superior portion of medial border of scapula	Elevation, downward rotation
Rhomboids (major and minor)	Under the trapezius, between the two scapulae	Major: spinous processes of T2–T5 Minor: spinous processes of C7–T1	Medial border of scapula	Retraction, downward rotation
Serratus anterior	Upper lateral side of the rib cage (deep)	Upper eight or nine ribs	Anterior aspect of medial border of scapula	Protraction, upper rotation
Pectoralis minor	Under the pectoralis major muscle on the anterior chest wall	Ribs 3, 4, and 5	Coracoid process of scapula	Protraction, depression, downward rotation

Muscles That Act on the Humerus (Figures 7–3 and 7–4; Table 7–4)

Together, the supraspinatus, infraspinatus, teres minor, and subscapularis muscles form the **rotator cuff** of the shoulder (the SITS muscles). This group of muscles provides movement for the shoulder joint as well as a great deal of stability. This explains why those suffering from rotator cuff injuries lack stability in the shoulder.

Shoulder flexors:
 Deltoid muscle (anterior portion)
 Pectoralis major muscle (clavicular head)
 Coracobrachialis muscle
 Biceps brachii muscle (short head)
Shoulder extensors:
 Latissimus dorsi muscle
 Teres major muscle
 Teres minor muscle
 Deltoid muscle (posterior portion)
 Infraspinatus muscle
 Pectoralis major muscle (sternal head)
 Triceps brachii muscle (long head)
Medial rotators:
 Deltoid muscle (anterior portion)
 Pectoralis major muscle
 Subscapularis muscle
 Teres major muscle
 Latissimus dorsi muscle
Shoulder abductors:
 Deltoid muscle (middle portion)
 Supraspinatus muscle
Horizontal abductors:
 Deltoid muscle (posterior portion)
 Teres minor muscle
 Infraspinatus muscle
Lateral rotators:
 Infraspinatus muscle
 Teres minor muscle
 Deltoid muscle (posterior portion)
Shoulder adductors:
 Pectoralis major muscle
 Coracobrachialis muscle
 Latissimus dorsi muscle
 Teres major muscle
Horizontal adductors:
 Pectoralis major muscle
 Coracobrachialis muscle
 Deltoid muscle (anterior portion)

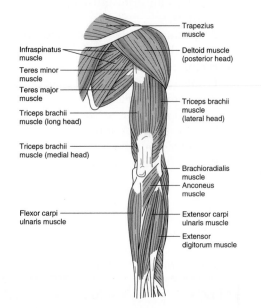

Figure 7–3. Posterior view of the muscles of the right arm.

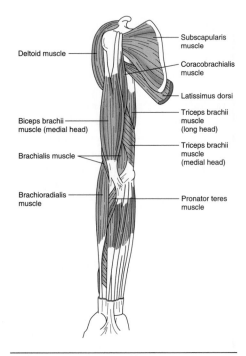

Figure 7–4. Anterior view of the muscles of the right arm.

Table 7–4. *Muscles that Act on the Humerus*

Muscle	Position	Origin	Insertion	Action
Supraspinatus	Above the spine of the scapula	Supraspinous fossa	Greater tubercle of the humerus	Abduction
Infraspinatus	Below the spine of the scapula	Infraspinous fossa	Greater tubercle of the humerus	External rotation, extension
Teres major	Below the infraspinatus muscle	Inferior angle of the scapula	Medial lip of the bicipital groove of the humerus	Extension, internal rotation, adduction
Teres minor	Between the infraspinatus and teres major muscles	Upper lateral border of the scapula	Greater tubercle of the humerus	Extension, external rotation
Subscapularis	Between the scapula and the rib cage	Subscapular fossa (anterior scapula)	Lesser tubercle of the humerus	Internal rotation
Latissimus dorsi	Middle to lower region of the back	Thoracolumbar aponeurosis from T7 to iliac crest (including the last three ribs)	Bicipital groove of the humerus	Extension, internal rotation, adduction
Pectoralis major (clavicular and sternal heads)	Superior portion of the anterior chest	Clavicular head: medial half of the clavicle Sternal head: sternum and cartilages of the first six ribs	Lateral lip of the bicipital groove of the humerus	Clavicular and sternal heads: adduction, horizontal adduction, internal rotation Clavicular head only: flexion Sternal head only: extension
Deltoids (anterior, middle, and posterior portions)	Over lateral aspect of the shoulder region	Anterior: lateral third of clavicle Middle: acromion process Posterior: spine of the scapula	Deltoid tuberosity on the humerus	Anterior: flexion, horizontal adduction, internal rotation Middle: abduction Posterior: extension, horizontal abduction, external rotation
Coraco-brachialis	Anterior armpit region	Coracoid process of the scapula	Middle of medial border of the humerus	Flexion, adduction, horizontal adduction

Muscles That Act on the Forearm (Table 7–5; see Figures 7–3 and 7–4)

The muscles of the forearm are not discussed in great detail, but here are some helpful hints on how to study these muscles. There are **six** main muscle groups in the forearm: the **flexor carpi, flexor digiti,** and **flexor pollicis** groups are all located on the anterior aspect of the forearm and the **extensor carpi, extensor digiti,** and **extensor pollicis** groups are all located on the posterior aspect of the forearm. The **carpi** groups all insert on the carpus and therefore flex and extend the wrist, the **digiti** groups insert on the digits and help flex and extend the fingers, and the **pollicis** groups insert on the **pollex** (thumb) and help flex and extend the thumb. Finally, words such as **longus** (long), **brevis** (short), **radialis, ulnaris, superficialis** (superficial), and **profundus** (deep) are used in the names of these muscles to indicate the relative lengths of the tendons of these

Table 7–5. *Muscles that Act on the Forearm*

Muscle	Position	Origin	Insertion	Action
Biceps brachii (long and short heads)	Anterior humerus	Long head: supraglenoid tubercle of the scapula Short head: coracoid process of the scapula	Radial tuberosity	Short head: elbow flexion, forearm supination, shoulder flexion
Brachialis	Lower, lateral humerus	Lower half of the anterolateral shaft of the humerus	Ulnar tuberosity	Elbow flexion
Triceps brachii (long, medial, and lateral heads)	Posterior humerus	Long head: infraglenoid tubercle of the scapula Medial head: posterior humerus Lateral head: superior, posterior humerus	Olecranon process of the ulna	All heads: elbow extension Long head only: shoulder extension
Anconeus	Posterolateral aspect of the elbow	Lateral epicondyle of the humerus	Olecranon process of the ulna	Elbow extension
Brachioradialis	Lateral forearm	Above lateral epicondyle of the humerus	Styloid process of the radius	Elbow flexion
Pronator teres	Anterior proximal forearm (deep)	Above medial epicondyle of the humerus	Midlateral shaft of the radius	Forearm pronation, elbow flexion
Pronator quadratus	Proximal to the wrist	Distal anterior ulna	Distal anterior radius	Forearm pronation
Supinator	Lateral aspect of the elbow (deep)	Below radial notch of the ulna	Anterior proximal radius	Forearm supination

muscles and their positions in the forearm. For example, the **flexor pollicis longus** is a long anterior muscle that flexes the thumb, the **extensor digitorum** is a posterior muscle that extends the fingers, the **flexor carpi ulnaris** is an anterior muscle on the ulnar side of the forearm that flexes the wrist, the **extensor carpi radialis longus** is a long posterior muscle on the radial side of the forearm that extends the wrist, and the **flexor digitorum superficialis** is an anterior superficial muscle that flexes the fingers.

Elbow flexors:
    Biceps brachii muscle
    Brachialis muscle
    Brachioradialis muscle
    Pronator teres muscle
Forearm supinators:
    Biceps brachii muscle
    Supinator muscle
Elbow extensors:
    Triceps brachii muscle
    Anconeus muscle
Forearm pronators:
    Pronator teres muscle
    Pronator quadratus muscle

Muscles of the Trunk and Back (Figures 7–5 and 7–6; Table 7–6)

Trunk flexors:
    Rectus abdominis muscle
    External oblique muscle
    Internal oblique muscle
Trunk extensors:
    Erector spinae muscles
Right trunk rotators:
    Left external oblique muscle
    Right internal oblique muscle
Left trunk rotators:
    Right external oblique muscle
    Left internal oblique muscle

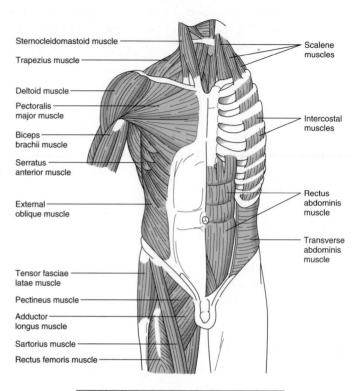

Figure 7–5. Anterior muscles of the trunk.

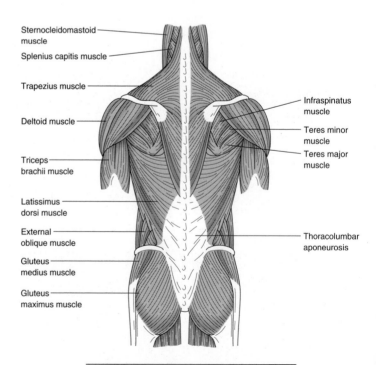

Figure 7–6. Posterior muscles of the trunk.

Table 7–6. *Muscles of the Trunk and Back*

Muscle	Position	Origin	Insertion	Action
Rectus abdominis	Anterior abdomen	Pubic spine	Costal cartilages for ribs 5, 6, and 7	Trunk (spine) flexion
External oblique	Lateral to the rectus abdominis muscle on the abdomen (superficial)	Lower eight ribs	Abdominal aponeurosis and iliac crest	Bilaterally: trunk flexion Unilaterally: lateral flexion, trunk rotation
Internal oblique	Under the external oblique muscle	Inguinal ligament and anterior iliac crest	Costal cartilages of the last four ribs and abdominal aponeurosis	Bilaterally: trunk flexion Unilaterally: lateral flexion, trunk rotation
Transverse abdominis	Under the internal oblique muscle (last layer of muscle in the abdomen)	Inguinal ligament, iliac crest, thoracolumbar aponeurosis, and lower margin of the rib cage	Abdominal aponeurosis	Compresses abdominal contents
Diaphragm	Between the thoracic and abdominal cavities	First three lumbar vertebrae, lower six costal cartilages, and xiphoid process	Central tendon (aponeurosis)	Increases the capacity of the thoracic cavity during inspiration
Erector spinae (spinalis, longissimus, and iliocostalis)	Runs longitudinally along the spine (deep) Spinalis: medial muscle Longissimus: middle muscle of the group Iliocostalis: lateral muscle	Spinalis: spinous processes of the cervical and thoracic vertebrae Longissimus: lumbar and thoracic transverse processes Iliocostalis: thoracolumbar aponeurosis	Spinalis: cervical and thoracic spinous processes and the occiput Longissimus: cervical and thoracic transverse processes and the mastoid process Iliocostalis: posterior ribs and cervical transverse processes	Bilaterally: trunk (spine) extension Unilaterally: lateral flexion
Quadratus lumborum	Deep to the erector spinae muscles in the low back, between the last ribs and ilium	Posterior iliac crest	12th rib and transverse processes of the lumbar vertebrae	Lateral flexion, hip elevation

Muscles of the Hip and Thigh (Figures 7–7 and 7–8; Table 7–7)

Hip flexors:
  Iliopsoas muscle
  Pectineus muscle
  Tensor fasciae latae muscle
  Rectus femoris muscle
  Sartorius muscle
  Adductor longus muscle
  Adductor brevis muscle
  Adductor magnus muscle
Hip abductors:
  Gluteus medius muscle
  Gluteus minimus muscle
  Iliopsoas muscle
  Tensor fasciae latae muscle
  Sartorius muscle
Hip extensors:
  Gluteus maximus muscle
  Biceps femoris muscle
  Semitendinosus muscle
  Semimembranosus muscle
Hip adductors:
  Pectineus muscle
  Adductor longus muscle
  Adductor brevis muscle
  Adductor magnus muscle
  Gracilis muscle
Hip lateral rotators:
  Gluteus maximus muscle
  Iliopsoas muscle
  Piriformis muscle
  Sartorius muscle
Hip medial rotators:
  Gluteus medius muscle
  Gluteus minimus muscle
  Tensor fasciae latae muscle
  Pectineus muscle
  Adductor longus muscle
  Adductor brevis muscle
  Adductor magnus muscle

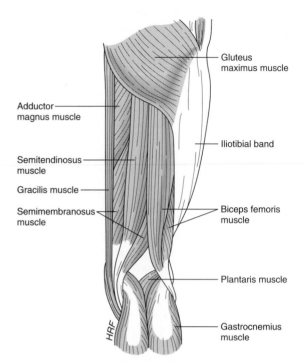

Figure 7–7. Posterior view of the thigh muscles on the right leg.

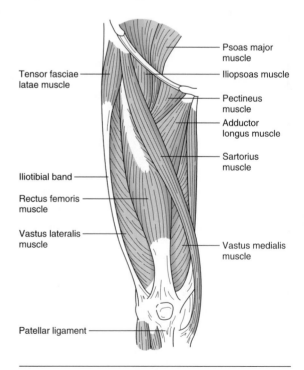

Figure 7–8. Anterior view of the thigh muscles on the right leg.

Table 7–7. *Muscles of the Hip and Thigh*

Muscle	Position	Origin	Insertion	Action
Gluteus maximus	Largest muscle in the gluteal region	Posterior ilium and sacrum	Gluteal tuberosity (on femur) and iliotibial tract	Hip extension, external rotation
Gluteus medius	Lateral hip	Lateral surface of the ilium	Greater trochanter of the femur	Hip abduction, internal rotation
Gluteus minimus	Under the gluteus medius muscle	Lateral surface of the lower ilium	Greater trochanter of the femur	Hip abduction, internal rotation
Piriformis	Under the gluteus maximus muscle	Anterior sacrum	Greater trochanter	External rotation
Tensor fasciae latae	Anterolateral hip	Anterior one third of the iliac crest	Tibia via the iliotibial tract	Hip abduction, hip flexion, internal rotation, and knee extension
Iliopsoas (psoas major and iliacus)	Deep in the abdominal cavity; becomes superficial in the inguinal region, then wraps around femur to insert	Psoas major: bodies of the lumbar vertebrae Iliacus: iliac fossa (internal surface of the ilium)	Lesser trochanter of the femur	Hip flexion, external rotation, and hip abduction
Sartorius	Crosses the thigh anteriorly	Anterior superior iliac spine Anterior body of pubis Rectus femoris: anterior inferior iliac spine Vastus lateralis: lateral lip of linea aspera Vastus intermedius: femoral shaft Vastus medialis: medial lip of linea aspera	Proximal medial shaft of the tibia (pes anserinus)	Hip flexion, external rotation, hip abduction, and knee flexion
Gracilis	Medial aspect of the thigh; runs next to adductors	Pectineal line (superior ramus of pubis)	Proximal medial shaft of the tibia (pes anserinus)	Hip adduction, knee flexion

(continued)

Table 7–7. *Muscles of the Hip and Thigh (Continued)*

Muscle	Position	Origin	Insertion	Action
Quadriceps femoris (rectus femoris, vastus lateralis, vastus intermedius, and vastus medialis muscles)	Anterior muscles of the thigh Rectus femoris: middle of anterior thigh Vastus lateralis: lateral thigh Vastus intermedius: under the rectus femoris Vastus medialis: medial thigh	Body of pubis and inferior ramus of pubis Rectus femoris: AIIS Vastus lateralis: lateral lip of linea aspera Vastus lateralis: anterior femur Vastus medialis: medial lip of linea aspera	Tibial tuberosity via the patellar tendon	Rectus femoris: hip flexion, knee extension Vastus muscles: knee extension
Pectineus	Anterior proximal aspect of the hip	Inferior ramus of pubis	Between the lesser trochanter and the linea aspera on the femur	Hip flexion, hip adduction, and internal rotation
Adductor longus	Anterior aspect of the medial thigh	Inferior ramus of pubis and ramus of ischium	Linea aspera on posterior femur	Hip adduction, hip flexion, and internal rotation
Adductor brevis	Middle of medial thigh		Linea aspera on posterior femur	Hip adduction, hip flexion, and internal rotation
Adductor magnus	Posterior aspect of medial thigh		Linea aspera on posterior femur	Hip adduction, hip flexion, and internal rotation
Hamstrings (biceps femoris, semitendinosus, and semimembranosus)	Biceps femoris: lateral posterior thigh Semitendinosus: middle posterior thigh Semimembranosus: medial posterior thigh	Biceps femoris: ischial tuberosity and linea aspera Semitendinosus: ischial tuberosity Semimembranosus: ischial tuberosity	Biceps femoris: head of fibula Semitendinosus: proximal medial shaft of the tibia (pes anserinus) Semimembranosus: posterior aspect of lateral condyle on the tibia	Hip extension, knee flexion

Muscles of the Lower Leg (Figures 7–9 and 7–10; Table 7–8)

The muscles of the lower leg are made up of four groups of three muscles each. The **triceps surae** group contains the two heads of the gastrocnemius muscle along with the soleus muscle and is found on the posterior calf. The **extensor** group contains the tibialis anterior, extensor hallucis longus, and extensor digitorum longus muscles and is found on the anterolateral aspect of the calf. The **peroneal** group (*perone = fibula*) contains the peroneus longus, peroneus brevis, and peroneus tertius muscles and surrounds the fibula on the lateral aspect of the calf. The **flexor** group contains the tibialis posterior, flexor digitorum longus, and flexor hallucis longus muscles and is found on the posteromedial aspect of the calf.

Knee flexors:
  Biceps femoris muscle
  Semitendinosus muscle
  Semimembranosus muscle
  Sartorius muscle
  Gracilis muscle
  Gastrocnemius muscle
  Plantaris muscle
  Popliteus muscle
Ankle plantar flexors:
  Gastrocnemius muscle
  Soleus muscle
  Plantaris muscle
  Tibialis posterior muscle
  Flexor digitorum longus muscle
  Flexor hallucis longus muscle
  Peroneus longus muscle
  Peroneus brevis muscle
Ankle invertors:
  Tibialis anterior muscle
  Tibialis posterior muscle
Knee extensors:
  Rectus femoris muscle
  Vastus lateralis muscle
  Vastus intermedius muscle
  Vastus medialis muscle
  Tensor fasciae latae muscle
Ankle dorsiflexors:
  Tibialis anterior muscle
    Extensor digitorum longus muscle
    Extensor hallucis longus muscle
  Peroneus tertius muscle
Ankle evertors:
  Peroneus longus muscle
    Peroneus brevis muscle
    Peroneus tertius muscle

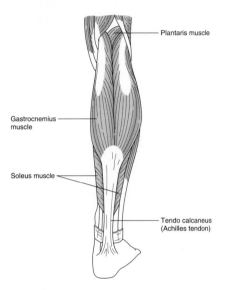

Figure 7–9. Posterior view of the lower leg muscles on the right leg.

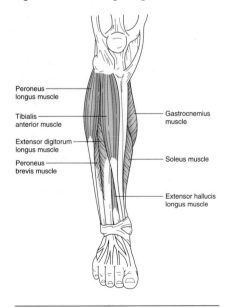

Figure 7–10. Anterior view of the lower leg muscles on the right leg.

Table 7–8. *Muscles of the Lower Leg*

Muscle	Position	Origin	Insertion	Action
Gastrocnemius	Superficial calf	Medial and lateral epicondyles of the femur	Calcaneus via the tendo calcaneus	Knee flexion, ankle plantar flexion
Soleus	Under the gastrocnemius muscle	Posterior tibia and fibula	Calcaneus via the tendo calcaneus	Ankle plantar flexion
Plantaris	Behind the knee; tendon lies between the gastrocnemius and soleus muscles	Lateral epicondyle of the femur	Calcaneus via the tendo calcaneus	Knee flexion, ankle plantar flexion
Popliteus	Behind the knee (deep)	Lateral condyle of the femur	Posterior proximal tibial shaft	Knee flexion
Tibialis anterior	Anterolateral lower leg	Anterolateral shaft of tibia	Base of 1st metatarsal and 1st cuneiform bones	Ankle dorsiflexion, ankle inversion
Extensor hallucis longus	Anterolateral lower leg, lateral to tibialis anterior	Anterior shaft of fibula and interosseous membrane	Base of 1st distal phalanx	Great toe extension, assists in ankle dorsiflexion
Extensor digitorum longus	Anterolateral lower leg, lateral to extensor hallucis longus	Proximal two thirds of anterior shaft of fibula	Dorsal surface of 2nd–4th middle and distal phalanges	Toe extension, assists in ankle dorsiflexion
Peroneus tertius	Lateral lower leg	Anterior distal fibula	Base of 5th metatarsal bone	Ankle eversion, ankle dorsiflexion
Peroneus longus	Lateral lower leg, posterior to peroneus tertius	Upper two thirds of lateral shaft of fibula	Base of 1st metatarsal bone and plantar surface of 1st cuneiform bone	Ankle eversion, assists in ankle plantar flexion
Peroneus brevis	Lateral lower leg, posterior to peroneus longus	Lower two thirds of lateral shaft of fibula	Base of 5th metatarsal bone	Ankle eversion, assists in ankle plantar flexion
Flexor hallucis longus	Posterior lower leg	Posterior shaft of fibula	1st distal phalanx	Great toe flexion, assists in ankle plantar flexion

(continued)

Table 7–8. *Muscles of the Lower Leg (Continued)*

Muscle	Position	Origin	Insertion	Action
Flexor digitorum longus	Posterior lower leg	Posterior shaft of tibia	Plantar surface of 2nd–4th distal phalanges	Toe flexion, assists in ankle plantar flexion
Tibialis posterior	Posterior to tibia and fibula	Posterior tibia and fibula	Navicular bone; 1st, 2nd, and 3rd cuneiform bones; cuboid bone; 2nd, 3rd, and 4th metatarsal bones	Ankle plantar flexion, ankle inversion

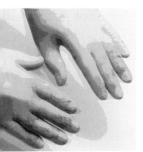

Chapter Eight

Nervous System

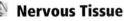

Nervous Tissue

Nerve Cells

As discussed in Chapter 3, there are two types of nerve cells: neurons and neuroglia.

Neurons — nerve cells responsible for conducting the action potential.
  Cell body — the main mass of the nerve cell; contains the nucleus.
  Dendrites — sensory receptors extending from the cell body; bring the action potential into the cell body.
  Axon — a long extension off of the cell body; responsible for conducting the action potential away from the cell body.
  Axon terminal — the far end of the axon; contains synaptic vesicles.
  Synaptic vesicles — tiny vesicles or sacs that contain the neurotransmitters produced by the neuron.
Neuroglia — supportive cells for the neurons in the central and peripheral nervous systems.
  Neurilemmocytes (Schwann cells) — cells that form the **myelin** sheath around the nerves of the peripheral nervous system.
  Nodes of Ranvier — tiny gaps in the myelin sheath at which the action potential is relayed along the neuron.
Nerve — a collection of nerve cells outside of the central nervous system.

> **Neurons** cannot mitotically divide to form new or additional neurons. Therefore, once dead, a neuron cannot be replaced. However, neurons can regenerate to allow a severed segment of the cell to grow back.

Nerve Impulse Transmission

Synapse — the space between a dendrite and a connecting axon terminal.
Neurotransmitters — hormones or chemical messengers contained and released by the synaptic vesicles; they stimulate or inhibit action potentials.

> **Myelin** is very important for the neurons of the peripheral nervous system. It protects the neuron itself, protects the action potential, and increases the action potential transmission rate. The nervous systems of infants are still growing myelin around the neurons. This helps explain why their motor movements are uncontrolled. As their myelin develops, their motor skills improve.

Epinephrine (adrenaline) — a sympathetic hormone released into the blood to prepare the body for "fight or flight."

Acetylcholine — a parasympathetic hormone released at the neuromuscular junction to initiate muscle contraction.

Divisions of the Nervous System

Central nervous system (CNS) — the main control center of the body; includes the **brain** and **spinal cord** only.

Peripheral nervous system (PNS) — includes all parts of the nervous system except the brain and spinal cord.

Somatic nervous system — nerves that control skeletal muscle contractions.

Autonomic nervous system — nerves that control smooth muscle, cardiac muscle, internal organs, and glands.

Sympathetic nervous system — prepares the body for stress; also called the "fight-or-flight" system.

Parasympathetic nervous system — prepares the body for rest; also called the "rest-and-digest" system.

Central Nervous System

Meninges — the three layers of tissue that surround the central nervous system.

Dura mater [dura = tough, hard; mater = mother] — the thickest, most external layer of the meninges.

Arachnoid membrane (mater) [arachnoid = spider web-like] — the delicate, web-like layer between the dura mater and pia mater; provides a space for the cerebrospinal fluid to circulate.

Pia mater [pia = soft, tender; mater = mother] — the thin, very vascular, innermost layer of the meninges; supports the blood vessels that supply nutrients to the brain.

Cerebrospinal fluid (CSF) — clear liquid formed in the ventricles of the brain that supports (or buoys up) the brain, cushions the central nervous system, and carries nutrients.

Brain (Figure 8–1)

Structure of the brain

Cerebrum — the superior portion of the brain; comprises about 80% of total brain mass; divided into right and left hemispheres by the longitudinal fissure; subdivided into lobes.

Gyri — the convoluted ridges or elevations in the cerebrum.

Sulci — the shallow grooves in the cerebrum.

Central sulcus — separates the frontal and parietal lobes.

Lateral sulcus — separates the parietal and temporal lobes.

Cerebellum — the second largest structure of the brain; found posterior and inferior to the cerebrum; also divided into hemispheres.

Brainstem — interconnects many nervous pathways and helps regulate many visceral functions.

Diencephalon — composed of the thalamus and hypothalamus.

Midbrain — found below the diencephalon.

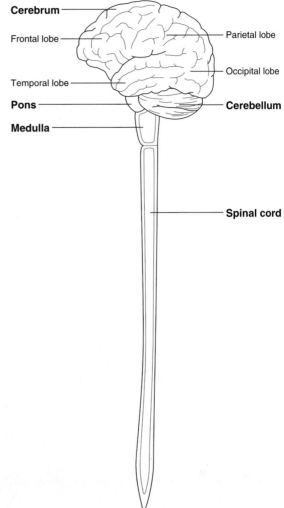

Figure 8–1. Main structures of the central nervous system.

Labels: Cerebrum, Frontal lobe, Temporal lobe, Pons, Medulla, Parietal lobe, Occipital lobe, Cerebellum, Spinal cord

Pons — rounded structure under the midbrain.

Medulla oblongata — enlarged portion of the brainstem directly above the spinal cord.

Ventricles — four pockets or spaces in the brain; cerebrospinal fluid is produced here.

Cerebrum

Right hemisphere — contains the sensory and motor pathways for the left side of the body; dominant for creativity, fantasy, art, and music appreciation.

Left hemisphere — contains the sensory and motor pathways for the right side of the body; dominant for logic, science, higher mathematics, languages, and verbal ideas.

The **lobes of the cerebrum** correspond in location to the bones of the skull.

Frontal lobe — responsible for personality, judgment, planning, and speech; contains the **motor cortex,** which initiates movement of skeletal muscles.

Parietal lobe — responsible for determining distance, size, and shape; contains the **sensory cortex,** which detects general sensory impulses from the skin (e.g., temperature, pain, texture).

Temporal lobe — contains the auditory and olfactory areas; stores memories of auditory and visual experiences.

Occipital lobe — contains the visual area for interpreting impulses from the retina of the eye.

Insular lobe — lies deep to the other four lobes; integrates cerebral activities; may also assist in memory.

Cerebellum

Functions include:

1. Coordination of voluntary muscles
2. Maintenance of balance
3. Maintenance of muscle tone

Brainstem

Diencephalon — composed of the thalamus and hypothalamus.
> **Thalamus** — sorts out incoming sensory impulses (except smell) and directs them to the proper areas of the cerebral cortex; also helps to filter out unimportant stimuli.
> **Hypothalamus** — controls the pituitary gland; regulates water and electrolyte balance, hunger, body temperature, sleep, sexual response, and emotions (e.g., anger, fear, pain, pleasure).

Midbrain — responsible for visual and auditory reflexes.

Pons — contains centers that control respiration.

Medulla oblongata — contains a cardiac control center, a vasomotor center, and a respiratory center.

Spinal Cord

Dorsal horns — gray matter in the spinal cord that extends posteriorly.

Ventral horns — gray matter in the spinal cord that extends anteriorly.

Reflex arc — the route followed by nerve impulses to provide a protective response to a potentially harmful stimulus.
> **Receptor organ** — the organ that contains the dendrites of the sensory neuron and receives the stimulus.
> **Afferent (sensory) neuron** — relays the action potential to the spinal cord.
> **Interneuron** — a short neuron in the central nervous system.
> **Efferent (motor) neuron** — conducts the action potential to the effector organ to elicit a response.
> **Effector organ** — the organ that produces or carries out a response; usually a skeletal muscle.

The spinal cord descends from the foramen magnum in the occipital bone down to about L1 and then divides into several portions collectively known as the **cauda equina** (tail of the horse). A **lumbar puncture** (insertion of a needle into the subarachnoid space to remove cerebrospinal fluid) is performed around L3 or L4, a few vertebrae below the end of the spinal cord.

Notice that the reflex arc does not involve the brain. Nervous impulses need only travel through the spinal cord (not the brain) to produce a response, thus saving valuable time. About the time the response has been produced, the brain is informed of what happened.

Peripheral Nervous System

Cranial nerves (Table 8–1)

There are 12 pairs of cranial nerves arising from the underside of the brain. Functions of the cranial nerves include:

In some reflex arcs (e.g., knee-jerk reflex) there is no interneuron. The afferent neuron synapses directly with the efferent neuron.

Table 8–1. *The Cranial Nerves*

Cranial Nerve	General Function	Specific Function
Olfactory (I)	SS	Smell
Optic (II)	SS	Sight
Oculomotor (III)	SM	Extrinsic muscles of the eye
Trochlear (IV)	SM	One extrinsic muscle of the eye (the superior oblique muscle)
Trigeminal (V)	GS and SM	GS: impulses from the forehead, upper jaw region, and lower jaw region SM: muscles of mastication
Abducens (VI)	SM	One extrinsic muscle of the eye (the superior oblique muscle)
Facial (VII)	SM and SS	SM: muscles of expression in the face SS: taste buds in the tongue
Vestibulocochlear (VIII)	SS	Hearing and equilibrium
Glossopharyngeal (IX)	SS, GS, and SM	SS: taste buds in the tongue GS: tongue SM: tongue
Vagus (X)	VM	Smooth muscle in visceral organs
Accessory (XI)	SM	Muscles of the head, neck, and shoulders
Hypoglossal (XII)	SM	Muscles of the tongue

GS = general sensory; SM = somatic motor; SS = special sensory; VM = visceral motor.

1. Special sensory (SS) [e.g., smell, taste, vision]
2. General sensory (GS) [e.g., pain, touch, temperature]
3. Somatic motor (SM) [voluntary movement]
4. Visceral motor (VM) [involuntary movement]

Spinal Nerves

There are 31 pairs of spinal nerves:

Cervical nerves (8 pairs)
Thoracic nerves (12 pairs)
Lumbar nerves (5 pairs)
Sacral nerves (5 pairs)
Coccygeal nerve (1 pair)

Dorsal root — the nerve root that protrudes posteriorly from the spinal cord.
  Dorsal root ganglion — collection of sensory nerve cell bodies outside of the dorsal root of the spinal cord.
Ventral root — the nerve root that protrudes anteriorly from the spinal cord.
Dermatome — the sensory area of the skin innervated by a particular spinal nerve root; follows a kind of "zebra-stripe" pattern on the skin.
Nerve plexus — a network of interconnecting nerves.
  Cervical plexus — arises from nerve roots C1 through C4 and a portion of C5; provides sensory innervation for the skin around the head, neck, and shoulders as well as motor innervation for some muscles in this same region.

There are many devices to help memorize the order of the cranial nerves. A modified version of the most famous jingle is:

On	→ Olfactory
Old	→ Optic
Olympus'	→ Oculomotor
Towering	→ Trochlear
Tops	→ Trigeminal
A	→ Abducens
Finn	→ Facial
And	→ Vestibulocochlear (formerly the auditory nerve)
German	→ Glossopharyngeal
Viewed	→ Vagus
A	→ Accessory
Hawk	→ Hypoglossal

Brachial plexus — arises from nerve roots C5 through T1 and is sometimes accompanied by portions of C4 and/or T2; provides sensory and motor innervation for the entire upper extremity and some neck muscles; gives rise to the axillary nerve, musculocutaneous nerve, radial nerve, median nerve, and ulnar nerve.

> The brachial plexus runs from the cervical region down through the armpit and into the arm. Trauma that affects either the neck or the upper arm and shoulder region can damage the brachial plexus, resulting in numbness, tingling, or paralysis down the arm and into the fingers.

Axillary nerve (C5 and C6) — sensory → lateral shoulder over the deltoid muscle; motor → deltoid and teres minor muscles.

Musculocutaneous nerve C5–C7) — sensory → lateral forearm; motor → biceps brachii, brachialis, and coracobrachialis muscles.

Radial nerve (C5–T1) — sensory → posterior forearm; motor → shoulder, elbow, wrist, and finger extensors, supinator muscle.

Median nerve — sensory → anterior side of fingers one through three and the lateral half of the fourth finger; motor → elbow, wrist, and finger flexors, pronators, and thenar eminence (anterior muscles of the thumb).

> The median nerve becomes compressed in **carpal tunnel syndrome.**

Ulnar nerve (C8–T1) — sensory → fifth finger and medial half of fourth finger; motor → intrinsic muscles of the hand.

> The ulnar nerve is often referred to as the "funny bone" as it runs under the medial epicondyle of the humerus.

Lumbosacral plexus — arises from nerve roots L1 through S4; provides sensory and motor innervation for the lower extremities; gives rise to the obturator nerve, femoral nerve, and sciatic nerve.

Obturator nerve (L2–L4) — sensory → upper medial thigh; motor → adductors and the gracilis muscle.

Femoral nerve (L2–L4) — sensory → anterior and lateral thigh; motor → quadriceps, iliopsoas, sartorius, and pectineus muscles.

Sciatic nerve (L4–S3) — sensory → posterior thigh; motor → hamstrings.

> The sciatic nerve divides just above the knee and becomes the **common peroneal nerve** and the **tibial nerve.** The common peroneal nerve comes around the lateral aspect of the lower leg just below the head of the fibula while the tibial nerve continues down the posterior calf. The tibial nerve further divides just below the medial malleolus into the **medial and lateral plantar nerves,** which innervate the skin and intrinsic muscles of the foot.

    Tibial nerve — sensory → posterior calf; motor → triceps surae muscle and flexors.

    Common peroneal nerve — sensory → anterior calf and dorsal surface of the foot; motor → extensors and the peroneal muscles.

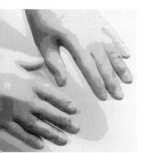

Chapter Nine

Sensory System

Vision—The Eye (Figure 9–1)

Anatomy of the Eye

Sclera — the outer white layer of the eye; the anterior portion becomes the cornea.
Cornea — the convex, clear part of the anterior sclera.
Choroid — the middle layer of the eye; contains large numbers of blood vessels.
Retina — the innermost layer of the eye; contains a pigmented, reflective layer and a layer of neurons (**rods** and **cones**) to detect light.
  Rods — neurons positioned in the peripheral areas of the retina that detect black and white.
  Cones — neurons concentrated within the **fovea centralis** (area of sharpest vision in the retina) that detect color.
Iris — the colored part of the eye; composed of smooth muscle; controls the amount of light that comes into the eye by dilating or constricting the pupil.
  Pupil — the space or opening in the iris.
Crystalline lens — a clear structure in the eye located between the iris and the vitreous humor; responsible for **accommodation** (adjustments to refract, or bend, the incoming light rays on the fovea centralis of the retina).

> Just as there is an area of most acute vision in the eye, there is also a blind spot. The small area where the optic nerve attaches to the eye contains no rods or cones; this area is referred to as the **optic disk.** To find the blind spot in your right eye, cover your left eye and stare closely at the dot. Then move your face toward or away from the paper until the cross disappears from view. (Your face should be about 10 inches from the page.)
>
> •   †

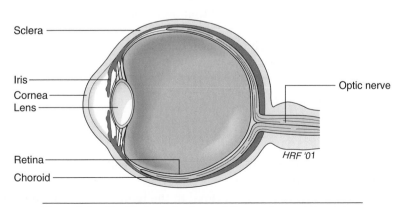

Figure 9–1. The internal structures of the eye from a lateral view.

Ciliary muscle — the circular muscle that surrounds the lens; responsible for adjusting the size of the lens in accommodation.

Suspensory ligament — a ligament made up of tiny fibers that connect the ciliary muscle to the lens.

Anterior chamber — the space between the cornea and the lens; filled with **aqueous humor.**

Vitreous chamber — the space behind the lens; filled with **vitreous humor and vitreous body.**

Extrinsic muscles — muscles used for eye movement.

> The **intrinsic muscles** in the eye are the **iris** and **ciliary muscle.** These muscles are under autonomic control to control the amount of incoming light and to help focus the light on the fovea centralis.

> **Superior rectus muscle** — rotates the eye upward and toward the midline.

> **Lateral rectus muscle** — rotates the eye away from the midline.

> **Inferior rectus muscle** — rotates the eye downward and toward the midline.

> **Medial rectus muscle** — rotates the eye toward the midline.

> **Superior oblique muscle** — rotates the eye downward and away from the midline.

> **Inferior oblique muscle** — rotates the eye upward and away from the midline.

Refractive Structures

Cornea
Aqueous humor
Lens
Vitreous humor and vitreous body

> As light enters the eye, cornea, aqueous humor, lens, and vitreous humor, all help to refract (bend) the light rays to focus the image onto the fovea centralis.

Protective Structures

Eyebrow and eyelashes — shade the eye and prevent particles and perspiration from falling into the eye.

Socket — forms a bony rim around the eye to protect against objects striking the eye.

Eyelid — a moveable covering for the eye that brushes off particles and moves tears over the surface of the eye to keep it moist.

Conjunctiva — the external lining that covers the anterior surface of the eyeball and the posterior surface of the eyelid; prevents particles from scratching the cornea and prevents objects (e.g., contact lenses) from moving posteriorly behind the eye.

Lacrimal apparatus — consists of the tear-producing glands and their ducts.

Lacrimal gland — an almond-shaped gland that secretes **lacrimal fluid** (tears) onto the upper lateral corner of the eye.

Nasolacrimal duct — a duct through the lacrimal bone that carries tears from the eye to the nasal cavity.

Hearing—The Ear (Figure 9–2)

External ear

Pinna (auricle) — the external portion of the ear; used to collect sound waves and direct them into the middle and inner ear.

External acoustic (auditory) meatus — a canal in the temporal bone through which the external ear canal runs.

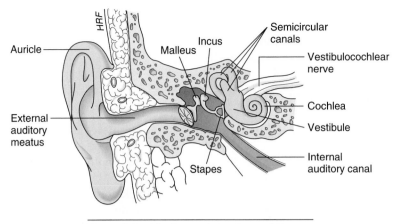

Figure 9–2. The internal structures of the ear.

Ceruminous glands — specialized wax-producing glands located in the tissue lining the external ear canal.

Tympanic membrane (eardrum) — detects sound waves.

Middle Ear

Ossicles — small bones of the middle ear; serve to amplify incoming sound waves.
  Malleus — hammer.
  Incus — anvil.
  Stapes — stirrup.
Auditory tube (eustachian tube) — a canal that connects the middle ear to the pharynx; used to equalize the pressure on both sides of the tympanic membrane.

> Sound waves are first detected by the tympanic membrane. The sound waves then travel from the malleus to the incus to the stapes and then into the inner ear.

Internal Ear

Cochlea [*cochlea = snail shell*] — the functional unit of hearing; contains the **organ of Corti.**
  Organ of Corti — the organ that transforms sound waves into nerve impulses.
Vestibule — the cavity in the inner ear that is sensitive to gravity and linear movement of the head.
Semicircular canals — the three bony canals that lie in each of the three cardinal planes; detect angular or rotational movement.

Smell—The Nose

Olfactory hairs — the sensitive portions of the **olfactory cells;** lie in the epithelial tissue of the nose.
Olfactory bulb — the structure positioned above the olfactory hairs; relays sensory information from the olfactory hairs to the **olfactory tract,** which is the first cranial nerve.

> The olfactory pathway goes like this: olfactory hairs → olfactory nerves → olfactory bulb → olfactory tract → temporal lobe of the cerebrum.

Taste—The Tongue and Mouth

Taste buds — receptors located mostly in the tongue that are sensitive to taste.

Sweet — on the tip of the tongue.
Sour — on the sides of the tongue.
Bitter — on the back of the tongue.
Salty — concentrated on the sides of the tongue.

Position—The Proprioceptors

Proprioceptors — specialized receptors found in joints, tendons, and muscles that sense body position.
Muscle spindles — found in muscles; provide information about the length or change in length of skeletal muscles.
Golgi tendon organ — an organ located where the muscle joins the tendon; protects the tendon by preventing excessive muscle tension from being applied to the tendon.

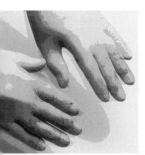

Chapter Ten

Endocrine System

Hormones

Hormones — chemical messengers of the body; made primarily from proteins and steroids.

Endocrine Glands (Figure 10–1)

Pituitary gland — a small gland situated beneath the hypothalamus in the brain; made up of two lobes (anterior and posterior); also called the "master gland."

> The **anterior pituitary and posterior pituitary** glands are each made up of separate and distinct tissue types. In size and shape they resemble two peas that have been pressed together.

    Anterior pituitary — produces growth hormone, thyroid-stimulating hormone, adrenocorticotropic hormone, prolactin, follicle-stimulating hormone, and luteinizing hormone.

        Growth hormone (GH) — controls the growth of bone and soft tissue; increases glycogen synthesis and fat metabolism in the body.

        Thyroid-stimulating hormone (TSH) — stimulates the thyroid gland to produce thyroid hormones for the regulation of metabolism.

        Adrenocorticotropic hormone (ACTH) — stimulates the growth and development of the adrenal cortex; stimulates the adrenal cortex to produce steroid hormones (e.g., cortisol).

        Prolactin (PRL) — stimulates the production of milk in the mammary glands of the breast; promotes breast development during pregnancy.

        Follicle-stimulating hormone (FSH) — stimulates development of the follicle (structure in the ovaries that produces the egg) in the female; stimulates the production of sperm in the male.

        Luteinizing hormone (LH) — acts with follicle-stimulating hormone to develop the follicle in the female; promotes ovulation in the female; stimulates the secretion of testosterone from the testes in the male.

    Posterior pituitary — produces antidiuretic hormone and oxytocin.

        Antidiuretic hormone (ADH) — increases water reabsorption in the kidneys to decrease urine formation; also called vasopressin.

        Oxytocin — stimulates contraction of the uterus in childbirth and milk let-down from the mammary glands of the breast.

Thyroid gland — a bowtie-shaped gland in the neck just below the larynx.

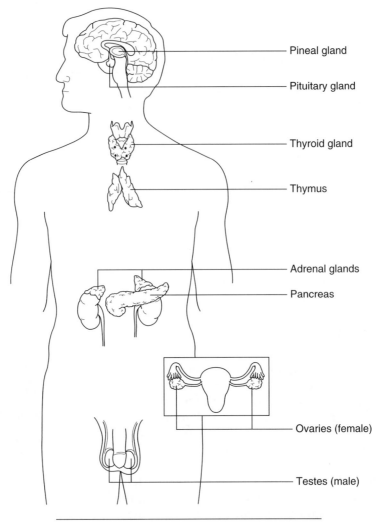

Figure 10–1. The major endocrine glands of the body.

Thyroxine (T_4) — increases the metabolic rate (e.g., catabolism of carbohydrates) and regulates the rate of growth; aided by another thyroid hormone called **triiodothyronine (T_3).**

Calcitonin — lowers blood calcium levels by inhibiting release of calcium from bone tissue.

Parathyroid glands — four to five tiny glands embedded in the posterior side of the thyroid gland.

    Parathyroid hormone — promotes calcium mobilization from bone tissue and calcium absorption from the intestines.

Pancreas — a long gland inferior to the stomach; contains the alpha, beta, and delta **pancreatic islet cells (islets of Langerhans),** which produce hormones.

    Insulin — a hormone (from the beta cells) that lowers blood sugar levels by promoting glucose uptake by the cells.

    Glucagon — a hormone (from the alpha cells) that increases blood sugar levels by various means (e.g., releasing glucose from glycogen stores in the liver).

Adrenal glands — pyramid-shaped glands located above the kidneys; also called suprarenal glands; divided into the cortex and medulla.

Adrenal cortex — produces cortisol, aldosterone, and sex hormones.
  Cortisol — released in response to stress; increases blood sugar levels, fatty acid immobilization, and immunosuppression.
  Aldosterone — helps regulate blood pressure by promoting sodium uptake and potassium secretion by the kidneys.
  Sex hormones — regulate sexual development(supplement the hormones produced by the gonads; see definition for gonads) and sex drive.
    Testosterone — causes masculinization.
    Estrogen — causes feminization.
    Progesterone — causes feminization.
Adrenal medulla — produces epinephrine and norepinephrine.
  Epinephrine — produces a sympathetic response (see Chapter 8).
  Norepinephrine — produces a sympathetic response slightly less intense than that produced by epinephrine.
Gonads — glands that produce sex cells (gametes) and sex hormones.
  Testes — the male gonads; produce testosterone.
    Testosterone — regulates the production of sperm cells in the testes and the development of the penis and accessory glands; causes development of male secondary sexual characteristics (e.g., body and facial hair, deeper voice, larger muscles and bones).
Ovaries — the female gonads; produce estrogen and progesterone.
  Estrogen — regulates menstrual changes and sex drive; responsible for the development of secondary sexual organs (e.g., mammary glands in breasts, vagina, uterine tubes) and female secondary sexual characteristics (e.g., fat deposition around hips and thighs, growth of breasts).
  Progesterone — develops the uterus in preparation for implantation of a fertilized egg; prevents spontaneous abortion of the fetus by preserving the lining of the uterus.
Thymus — an organ found in the mediastinum above the heart that produces **T cells** (thymus-dependent cells), specialized lymphocytes used in body immunity.
  Thymosin — stimulates the T cells in the body that have already been produced by the thymus.
Pineal gland — a small gland found in the midbrain of the brainstem.
  Melatonin — regulates sleep–wake cycles of the body.

Other Hormone-Producing Organs

Kidneys — major function involves filtering the blood and producing urine (see Chapter 15); also produce hormones.
  Renin — stimulates an increase in water retention by the body, thus increasing blood pressure.
  Erythropoietin — stimulates the production of red blood cells by the red bone marrow.
Placenta — an organ responsible for regulating gas, nutrient, waste, and hormonal exchange between the mother and fetus during pregnancy.
  Human chorionic gonadotropin (HCG) — simulates the action of luteinizing hormone, growth hormone, and prolactin.

> **Human chorionic gonadotropin** is the hormone detected in the urine by home pregnancy tests.

Stomach — a major organ of the digestive system; secretes hormones that stimulate the gallbladder and pancreas, promote digestion, and inform the brain when you have eaten enough.

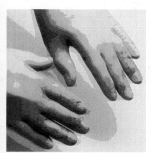

Chapter Eleven

Cardiovascular System

Blood

Functions of Blood

1. **Transports** gases (e.g., oxygen, carbon dioxide), nutrients (building blocks) to the tissues, waste products from the tissues, and hormones.
2. **Regulates** the pH of the body, the amount of fluids in the tissues (by maintaining a proper osmotic pressure), and body temperature.
3. **Protects** against pathogens and blood loss.

Blood Constituents (Figure 11–1)

Blood plasma — the liquid portion of unclotted blood.
    Plasma proteins — proteins found in the plasma; include albumins (help regulate blood pressure), globulins (help with transport and immunity), and fibrinogen (assists in blood clotting).
Blood serum — the liquid portion of clotted blood; plasma that has had the fibrinogen and other clotting factors removed so that the blood clotting function is minimized.
Formed elements — the blood cells and platelets carried by the plasma.

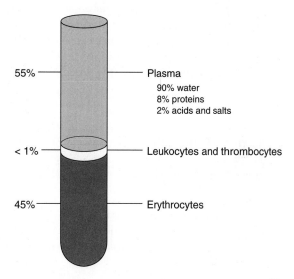

Figure 11–1. The elements of the blood when they are separated.

Erythrocytes (red blood cells) — biconcave, disk-shaped cells that do not contain nuclei; constitute approximately 40% to 50% of whole blood, depending on gender; have a life span of approximately 120 days.

Hemoglobin — an oxygen-carrying molecule made from iron; found in the erythrocytes.

Leukocytes (white blood cells) — cells responsible for the body's defenses; contain nuclei and have varied life spans.

Thrombocytes (platelets) — cell fragments without nuclei that assist in blood clotting; have a life span of approximately 8 to 10 days.

> The red blood cell count (i.e., the percentage of whole blood that is actually red blood cells) is referred to as the **hematocrit** [*hemo = blood; crit = count*]. This number differs in men and women (40% to 52% for men and 37% to 47% for women), probably due to metabolism, menstruation, and iron storage differences.

Blood Clotting

Hemostasis [*hemo = blood; stasis = stay*] — the process of blood clotting; starts with muscle contraction in response to injury, proceeds to formation of a platelet plug, and ends with formation of a blood clot.

1. **Contraction**—smooth muscle of the blood vessel constricts when damaged or cut.
2. **Platelet plug**—platelets in the region of damage become sticky and bind together with other platelets, blood cells, and the walls of the vessel.
3. **Blood clot**—**prothrombin** is converted into **thrombin**, **fibrinogen** into **fibrin** (a thread-like protein), and the fibrin threads form the clot.

> There are five kinds of leukocytes that all share the same basic function of defending the body against foreign invaders. These cells have the ability to squeeze through tiny pores in capillary walls and escape into the tissues, which is a process called **diapedesis**. One kind of white blood cell is called a **macrophage** [*macro = big; phago = to eat*] or "big eater."

Blood Typing

Antigen — a protein bound to the surface of a cell (e.g. antigens A, B, Rh, M, N); gives the cell identity.

Antibody (immunoglobulin) — a component of the immune system that attaches to a specific antigen on a cell; binds cells with other similar cells (**opsonization**), which prepares the cells for phagocytosis; the body produces antibodies only for foreign antigens.

Blood transfusion — infusion of red blood cells into a living body; requires blood typing to match the recipient with an appropriate donor (Table 11–1).

> The **clotting factors** prothrombin, thrombin, fibrinogen, and fibrin are the last of the clotting factors to get activated. There are actually 11 other clotting factors that have to be activated before prothrombin can be converted to thrombin. It is like a domino effect that becomes amplified at each step. A deficiency of any one of these factors leads to **hemophilia**.

The Heart

Structure of the Heart (Figure 11–2)

Tissues of the heart

Endocardium — the inner layer of the heart; composed of epithelial and connective tissues.

Myocardium — the thick middle layer of the heart; composed of **cardiac muscle tissue** that contracts regularly.

> When a patient needs a blood transfusion, it is best to give him blood that is his same type. However, in the event that the patient's blood type is not available, other suitable types may be substituted. Precaution must be taken not to give an individual any blood cells that carry foreign antigens. Type O Rh-negative is the **universal donor** because it carries no antigens. Type AB Rh-positive is the **universal recipient** because it carries all of the antigens.

Table 11–1. *Blood Types*

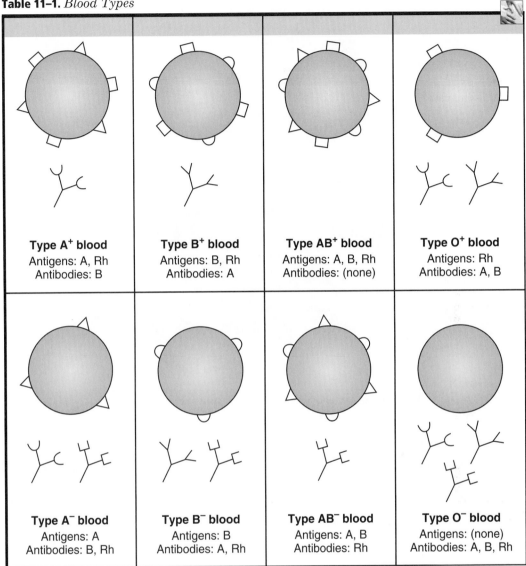

Type A⁺ blood Antigens: A, Rh Antibodies: B	**Type B⁺ blood** Antigens: B, Rh Antibodies: A	**Type AB⁺ blood** Antigens: A, B, Rh Antibodies: (none)	**Type O⁺ blood** Antigens: Rh Antibodies: A, B
Type A⁻ blood Antigens: A Antibodies: B, Rh	**Type B⁻ blood** Antigens: B Antibodies: A, Rh	**Type AB⁻ blood** Antigens: A, B Antibodies: Rh	**Type O⁻ blood** Antigens: (none) Antibodies: A, B, Rh

*Blood type AB Rh-positive is the universal recipient blood. †Blood type O Rh-negative is the universal donor blood.

Epicardium — the outer covering or membrane around the heart; composed mostly of connective tissue.

Pericardium — the loose-fitting sac around the heart; composed of serous membranes.

Heart chambers

Right atrium — the upper right chamber; receives deoxygenated blood from the body.

Right ventricle — the lower right chamber; pumps blood to the lungs.

Left atrium — the upper left chamber; receives oxygenated blood from the lungs.

Left ventricle — the lower left chamber; pumps blood to the body.

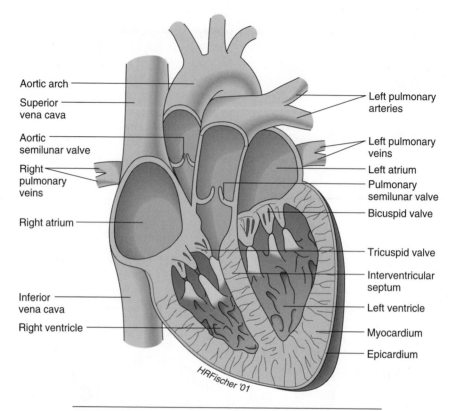

Figure 11–2. Anterior view of the major structures of the heart.

Partitions in the heart

Interatrial septum — the partition between the two atria; composed mostly of fibrous tissue.

Interventricular septum — the partition between the two ventricles; composed mostly of myocardium.

Heart Valves

Atrioventricular (AV) valves — the valves that separate the atria and ventricles.
> **Tricuspid valve** — separates the right atrium and the right ventricle.
> **Bicuspid (mitral) valve** — separates the left atrium and the left ventricle.

Semilunar valves — the valves that separate the ventricles from the blood vessels that attach to them.
> **Pulmonary semilunar valve** — separates the right ventricle from the pulmonary trunk.
> **Aortic semilunar valve** — separates the left ventricle from the aorta.

Tremendous pressure develops against the atrioventricular valves when the ventricles contract. Therefore, the cusps of these valves have small tendons called **chordae tendineae** that keep them from being blown out, as a strong wind would blow out an umbrella.

The two **heart sounds**—"lubb" and "dubb"—are produced when one set of valves closes. "Lubb," the louder of the two sounds, occurs as the atrioventricular valves close. The softer "dubb" sound occurs as the semilunar valves close.

Contraction of the Heart

Cardiac cycle — the cycle involving periods of **systole** (contraction of myocardium) and **diastole** (relaxation of myocardium) to fill and empty the chambers of the heart (Table 11–2).

Conduction pathway of the heart — specialized strands of cardiac muscle tissue that coordinate the rhythmic contractions of the heart.

  Sinoatrial (SA) node — acts as the "pacemaker" of the heart; situated in the posterior wall of the right atrium.

  Atrioventricular (AV) node — the relay point for impulses coming from the sinoatrial node; situated toward the bottom of the interatrial septum.

  Atrioventricular bundle (bundle of His) — short bundle of fibers at the top of the interventricular septum that relay the nervous impulse from the atrioventricular node to the left and right ventricles.

  Bundle branches — two branches that extend from the atrioventricular bundle and bring the impulse down the interventricular septum.

  Purkinje fibers — small fibers at the ends of the bundle branches that connect to and stimulate the contraction of the myocardium.

Cardiac output — the volume of blood pumped out of the heart per minute (usually measured in L/min); calculated by multiplying the stroke volume of the heart by the heart rate.

> **Cardiac output** changes dramatically in an individual depending on the activity being performed. At rest, normal cardiac output ranges between 4.5 and 5.5 L/min. During exercise, heart rate and stroke volume both increase, elevating the cardiac output to as high as 25 L/min.

  Stroke volume — the volume of blood pumped out of the left ventricle every time it contracts (measured in L/beat).

  Heart rate — the number of times the ventricles contract per minute (measured in beats/min).

Blood Flow Through the Heart (Figure 11–3)

Blood Supply of the Heart

Coronary arteries — blood vessels that take blood to the heart tissue.
Coronary veins — blood vessels that drain the heart tissue.
Coronary sinus — collects blood from the coronary veins.

Table 11–2. *The Phases of the Cardiac Cycle*

Phase	Ventricles	Atria	AV Valves	Semilunar Valves	Movement of Blood
1	Diastole	Diastole	Open	Closed	Blood filling atria and ventricles
2	Diastole	Systole	Remain open	Closed	Blood fills ventricles completely
3	Systole	Diastole	Close (causes "lubb" sound)	Open	Blood pumped from ventricles out of the heart
4	Diastole	Diastole	Open	Close (causes "dubb" sound)	Blood filling atria

AV = atrioventricular.

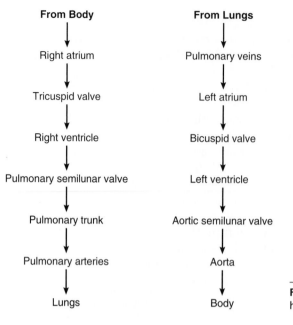

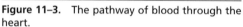

Figure 11–3. The pathway of blood through the heart.

Heart Rates

Bradycardia — slow heart rate (i.e., below 60 beats/min).
Tachycardia — fast heart rate (i.e., above 100 beats/min).

Blood Vessels

Classifications

Arteries — blood vessels that carry blood away from the heart.
    Arterioles — small arteries.
Veins — blood vessels that carry blood toward the heart.
    Venules — small veins.
Capillaries — small blood vessels that connect arterioles and venules; where exchange of gases, nutrients, wastes, and hormones takes place.

Systems

Pulmonary vessels — all of the blood vessels that carry blood to and from the lungs.
Systemic vessels — all of the blood vessels that carry blood to and from the body.

Histology of Blood Vessels (Table 11–3)

Tunica externa [*tunic = coat; externa = outer*] — external layer of connective tissue.
Tunica media [*media = middle*] — middle layer made up of smooth muscle tissue.
Tunica intima [*intima = internal*] — layer of squamous epithelial tissue (often called the endothelium) that lines the lumen.
Lumen — cavity in the vessel through which the blood flows.

Table 11–3. *Comparison of Arteries and Veins*

Arteries	Veins
Carry blood away from the heart	Carry blood toward the heart
Thick tunica media	Thin tunica media
Do not contain one-way valves	Contain one-way valves
Low degree of variance in position and distribution	High degree of variance in position and distribution
Positioned deep	Positioned superficial and deep
High pressure	Low pressure
Fast blood flow	Slow blood flow
Blood pumped by heart	Blood pumped by skeletal muscles

Systemic Vessels

The following list includes the major arteries and veins of the body and the hepatic portal system. Refer to the drawings provided and your own body while studying the blood vessels to understand their position in relation to other structures (e.g., muscles, bones, nerves, organs).

Arteries (Figure 11–4)

Aorta
    Ascending aorta
    Arch of the aorta
    Descending aorta
Brachiocephalic trunk
    Right common carotid artery
    Right subclavian artery
Common carotid artery
Internal carotid artery
External carotid artery
Subclavian artery
Axillary artery
Brachial artery
Radial artery
Ulnar artery
Celiac trunk
    Left gastric artery
    Common hepatic artery
    Splenic artery
Superior mesenteric artery
Renal artery
Gonadal arteries
Inferior mesenteric artery
Common iliac artery
External iliac artery
Internal iliac artery
Femoral artery
Popliteal artery
Anterior tibial artery
Posterior tibial artery

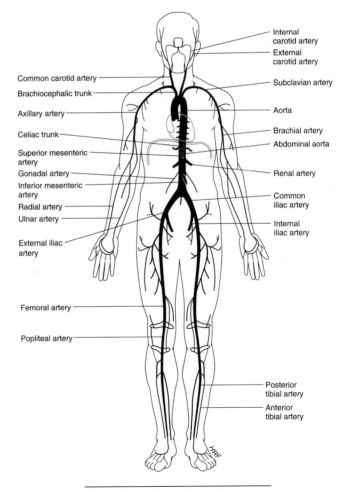

Figure 11–4.   The arteries of the body.

Veins (Figure 11–5)

Superior vena cava
Brachiocephalic vein
Jugular veins
Subclavian vein
Axillary vein
Brachial veins
Radial veins
Ulnar veins
Cephalic vein
Basilic vein
Median cubital vein
Inferior vena cava
Hepatic veins
Renal veins
Gonadal veins
Common iliac vein
External iliac vein
Internal iliac vein
Femoral vein
Saphenous veins
Popliteal vein
Anterior tibial veins
Posterior tibial veins

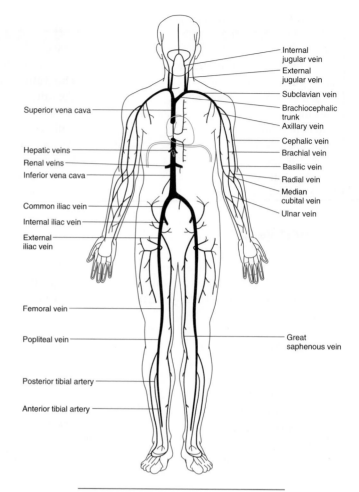

Figure 11–5. The major veins of the body.

Hepatic Portal System (Figure 11–6)

Hepatic portal vein
Splenic vein
Gastric vein
Superior mesenteric vein
Inferior mesenteric vein

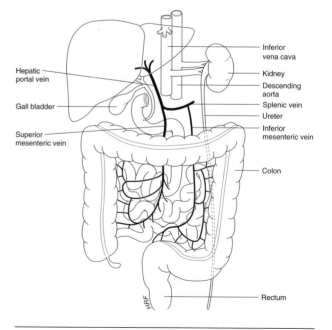

Figure 11–6. The major blood vessels in the hepatic portal system.

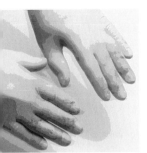

Chapter Twelve

Lymphatic and Immune Systems

Lymphatic System

Lymph

Lymph fluid (lymph) — the name given to the fluid that enters into the lymphatic vessels.

Lymph fluid, or **lymph,** has almost the same composition as blood plasma. In fact, lymph fluid begins as blood plasma that filters out of the capillary walls because the mechanical pressure pushing fluid out of the capillary is greater than the osmotic pressure pulling the fluid back in. Without the lymph vessels to take this excess fluid away, **edema** (swelling) would result.

Lymphatic Vessels (Figure 12–1)

Lymph capillaries — smallest, microscopic vessels of the lymphatic system; walls are composed of squamous epithelium to readily allow fluid to enter.

Right lymphatic duct — brings lymph from the upper right quadrant of the body and drains into the right subclavian vein.

Thoracic duct — brings lymph from the upper left quadrant and lower extremities of the body and drains into the left subclavian vein.

    Cisterna chyli — a sac-like enlargement on the inferior portion of the thoracic duct.

Lacteals — small, specialized lymph vessels in the villi of the small intestine that carry lymph fluid and fat, a combination referred to as **chyle** (see Chapter 14).

Lymphoid Organs

Lymphoid organs — organs that help to remove impurities (e.g., bacteria, dead cells, cancer cells) and process lymphocytes.

    Lymph nodes — patches of lymphoid tissue that contain high amounts of phagocytes and produce lymphocytes; usually occur in clusters and carry the name of the region of the body in which they are found; some of the major lymph nodes in the body include those in Figure 12–1:

        Axillary lymph nodes
        Parotid lymph nodes
        Iliac lymph nodes
        Cervical lymph nodes
        Mesenteric lymph nodes
        Inguinal lymph nodes

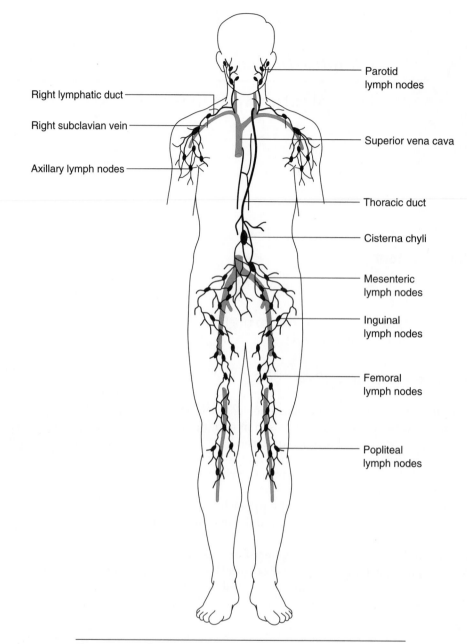

Figure 12–1. The major lymph nodes and lymph vessels in the body.

Mandibular lymph node
Lumbar lymph nodes
Popliteal lymph nodes

Spleen — fist-sized organ found beneath the diaphragm on the left side of the body, under the 11th and 12th ribs; functions of the spleen include:

1. Filtering the blood
2. Producing red blood cells before birth
3. Destroying old, worn out red blood cells
4. Acting as a reservoir for blood storage in case of hemorrhage

Tonsils — three pairs of lymphoid organs found in the pharynx (throat); help to fight infection and filter the blood.

    Pharyngeal tonsils ("adenoids") — located just below the nasopharynx.

    Palatine tonsils — visible on the walls of the oropharynx when looking into the mouth.

    Lingual tonsils — located on the posterior aspect of the tongue.

Thymus — lymphoid organ found in the mediastinum above the heart; produces **thymosin,** a hormone that converts white blood cells into **T lymphocytes,** which are essential in activation of the immune system.

> When young, our bodies are still building immunity to the diseases that surround us; therefore, the **thymus** is larger and more active. After adolescence, our immunity is largely in place, so the thymus decreases in size and activity.

Immune System

Nonspecific Immunity

Nonspecific immunity — defenses of the body that do not discriminate between one threat and another; nonspecific defenses include:

Physical barriers (e.g., skin, hair, mucus, earwax, tears, sweat)

Phagocytes (e.g., mobile and free macrophages)

Reflexes (e.g., coughing, sneezing, vomiting, diarrhea, fever)

Inflammation

Complement (destroys foreign cell walls)

Interferon (interferes with virus replication)

Normal flora (e.g., the normal population of bacteria that inhabit the skin and gastrointestinal tract, preventing harmful bacteria from residing and multiplying in the body)

Specific Immunity

Specific immunity — immunity produced by lymphatic tissue and immune cells; results from exposure to a specific antigen from a foreign cell.

Components of specific immunity

Antibodies (immunoglobulins) — attach to a specific antigen; bind similar cells together (a process called **opsonization**), which prepares the cells for phagocytosis.

T lymphocytes (T cells) — specialized white blood cells that originate from the thymus; responsible for activating and regulating the body's immune response.

    T helper cells — cells responsible for identifying an antigen as foreign and initiating defense mechanisms (e.g., the production of antibodies) to defend against it.

    T cytotoxic cells — cells capable of directly identifying a foreign antigen on the surface of a cell, binding to it, and destroying the cell.

B cells — specialized lymphocytes responsible for identifying a foreign antigen and differentiating into **plasma cells** to produce antibodies for that antigen.

    Memory cells — B cells that remain in the body for years after the first exposure to an antigen to provide protection in the event of a subsequent exposure.

Types of specific immunity

Inborn immunity — immunity dependent on species, race, and individuality.

Acquired immunity — immunity that develops after exposure to a foreign antigen.

Active naturally acquired immunity — immunity acquired by actual exposure to the foreign antigen by natural means (e.g., catching chickenpox).

Passive naturally acquired immunity — immunity from antibodies inherited from the mother through the placenta or through breast milk.

Active artificially acquired immunity — immunity developed after inoculation of a foreign antigen in a vaccine or in a killed or attenuated toxoid.

Passive artificially acquired immunity — immunity from antibodies taken from one individual and given to another (e.g., gamma globulin shots).

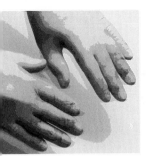

Chapter Thirteen

Respiratory System

Divisions of the Respiratory System

Upper Respiratory Tract (Figure 13–1)

Nasal cavities — two spaces separated by a bony partition called the **nasal septum;** found between the eyes, above the oral cavity.
  Nostrils — the two openings into the nasal cavities.
  Nasal choana or conchae [*choana = funnel*] — curved projections along the lateral sides of the nasal cavities; filter out dust particles and warm and humidify the incoming air.
  Sinuses — small cavities in the bones of the skull; lined with mucous membranes; communicate with the nasal cavities.
Pharynx [*pharynx = throat*] — passageway lined with mucous membranes; connects the nasal cavities to the larynx.

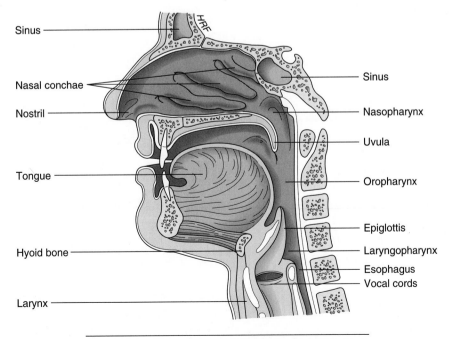

Figure 13–1. The structures of the upper respiratory tract.

Nasopharynx — the uppermost portion of the pharynx; lies directly behind the nasal cavities; contains the **pharyngeal tonsils** (adenoids).

Oropharynx — the middle portion of the pharynx; lies directly behind the oral cavity; contains the **palatine tonsils** (on the walls of the oropharynx) and the **lingual tonsils** (posterior aspect of the tongue) [see Chapter 12].

> The nasopharynx is used for respiratory function only, while the oropharynx and laryngopharynx are used for both respiratory and digestive functions.

Laryngopharynx — the bottom portion of the pharynx; lies directly above the larynx.

Larynx [*larynx = upper windpipe*] — a cartilaginous structure; contains the **vocal cords;** contains a small protrusion of cartilage commonly called the Adam's apple; also called the "voice box."

Glottis — the opening between the two vocal cords.

Epiglottis — a cartilaginous structure above the glottis; folds down over the glottis during swallowing to prevent food and water from entering the trachea.

Lower Respiratory Tract (Figure 13–2)

Trachea — a rigid tube made up of a series of horseshoe-shaped cartilaginous rings; connects the pharynx to the bronchi of the lungs; also called the "windpipe."

Lungs — organs in which gas exchange takes place.

Mediastinum — anatomical space between the two lungs where the trachea, heart, major blood vessels, and esophagus are found.

Bronchi — cartilaginous tubes that extend from the trachea into the lungs.

> Remember that exchange of gases in the lungs takes place by **diffusion.** The gases move spontaneously from an area of high concentration to an area of low concentration.

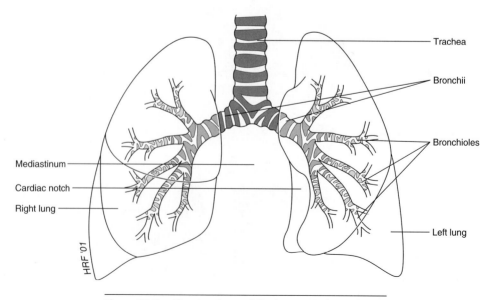

Figure 13–2. The structures of the lower respiratory tract.

Bronchioles — small bronchi.
Terminal bronchioles — the last segments of the
bronchioles; connect to the alveoli.
Alveoli — tiny sacs that number about 350 million per
lung; where gas exchange takes place.
Surfactant — a lipid secreted in the alveoli; reduces
the surface tension of the water within the lung,
thus decreasing the energy required to fill the
alveoli with air.
Pleural membranes — serous membranes associated
with the lungs; produce a lubricant to reduce friction
between the lungs and the walls of the pleural
cavity.
Parietal pleura — serous membrane surrounding the
internal walls of the thoracic cavity.
Visceral pleura — serous membrane lining the outer
surfaces of the lungs.

> The left lung has a **cardiac notch** to accommodate the heart; therefore, the left lung is smaller and has only two lobes while the right lung has three lobes.

> Premature babies commonly experience respiratory problems because they are born before their lungs have started to produce **surfactant.** Without surfactant, they must use a tremendous amount of energy (sometimes as much as 30% of their metabolic energy versus approximately 3% to 5% normally) to overcome the surface tension of the water in their lungs and fill their lungs with air.

Physiology of Respiration

Phases of Breathing

Inhalation — active phase of breathing in which energy is
used to draw air into the lungs.
Exhalation — passive phase of breathing in which air is
pushed out of the lungs.

> During **inhalation,** the diaphragm contracts and flattens. This action, along with the contractions of other muscles of respiration, increases the size of the thoracic cavity, drawing air into the lungs. During **exhalation** these muscles relax, allowing the thoracic cavity to resume its original capacity, thus pushing the air out of the lungs.

Lung Volumes and Capacities

Tidal volume — the volume of air moved in or out of the
lungs in one breath during quiet, relaxed breathing;
approximately 0.5 L.
Residual volume — the volume of air that remains in the
lungs after maximum exhalation; approximately 1.2 L.
Vital capacity — the volume of air that can be exhaled after maximum inhalation;
approximately 4.8 L.
Total lung capacity — the total volume of air that can be contained in the lungs;
approximately 6 L.

Muscles of Respiration

The following is a list of the muscles used in respiration.
Please refer to Chapter 7 for a detailed description of the position, origin, insertion, and specific action of each muscle.

Inhalation
Diaphragm (controls most of quiet, relaxed inhalation)
External intercostal muscle
Scalene muscles
Sternocleidomastoid muscle

> Damage to the upper cervical spine can cause damage to the **phrenic nerve,** the nerve that comes from nerve roots C3–C5 and innervates the diaphragm. This explains why those who suffer from damage to the first three or four cervical vertebrae often need ventilators to help them breathe while those who injure cervical vertebrae below C3 or C4 can usually breathe on their own.

Exhalation
Internal intercostal muscle
External oblique muscle
Internal oblique muscle
Transversus abdominis muscle

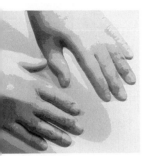

Chapter Fourteen

Digestive System

Divisions of the Digestive System

Digestive (gastrointestinal) tract — the continuous pathway that food follows from the mouth to the anus.

Accessory organs — organs that secrete substances that travel through ducts into the digestive tract to help with digestion; not a part of the digestive tract.

Digestive (Gastrointestinal) Tract (Figure 14–1)

Walls of the Digestive Tract

Serosa — the external epithelial membrane that surrounds the organs (**visceral peritoneum**) and walls (**parietal peritoneum**) in the **peritoneal cavity** (abdominal cavity).

> **Mesentary** — a supportive structure composed of two layers of serosa; connects to the intestines; contains the blood vessels, lymph vessels, and nerves that run to and from the intestinal wall.

Muscularis — two layers of smooth muscle (circular and longitudinal); mixes food with digestive juices and moves food through the digestive tract.

> **Peristalsis** — the wave-like movement of food through the digestive tract.

Submucosa — the layer of connective tissue beneath the mucosa that contains blood vessels, nerves, and lymph vessels.

Mucosa — internal mucous membrane through which the body absorbs digested substances into the blood.

> **Villi** — small, finger-like projections on the mucosa where absorption of nutrients and fats takes place; contain blood vessels and **lacteals** (specialized lymph vessels) [see Chapter 12].

Regions of the Digestive Tract

Oral cavity (mouth) — the beginning of the digestive tract; aids in speech, **ingests** (takes in) food, and prepares food for digestion by breaking it up into smaller pieces.

> **Salivary glands** — three pairs of **accessory organs to the digestive system;** produce **saliva,** a fluid that helps break down starches into sugars.

>> **Parotid glands** — the largest pair of salivary glands; located anterior and inferior to the ear.

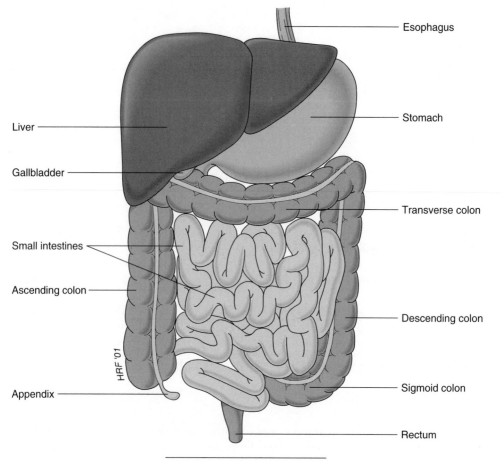

Figure 14–1. The digestive tract.

Submandibular glands — salivary glands located under the mandible.

Sublingual glands — salivary glands located under the tongue.

Pharynx (throat) — divided into the **oropharynx** and the **laryngopharynx;** a passageway for food; also used for respiration.

Soft palate — soft tissue on the back of the roof of the mouth; contains the **uvula** (a fleshy, V-shaped mass).

Esophagus — a muscular tube that carries food from the pharynx to the stomach.

Cardiac sphincter — a circular or ring-shaped muscle at the base of the esophagus; prevents food and gastric juice from going back up into the esophagus.

> When swallowing (a process called **deglutition**), a small portion of chewed food together with saliva is called a **bolus.**

Stomach — a J-shaped organ positioned in the left upper abdomen.

Fundus of the stomach — the bulge at the top of the stomach.

Rugae — folds in the stomach lining.

Pylorus — the lowest portion of the stomach; contains the pyloric sphincter.

> Sometimes food and gastric juice slips through the cardiac sphincter and reenters the esophagus, causing the irritation or burning we call **heartburn.**

Pyloric sphincter — a muscle that controls the passage of food from the stomach into the small intestine.

Gastric juice — the acidic fluid (pH around 2.1) produced by the stomach; contains **hydrochloric acid** and **pepsin,** an enzyme that breaks down proteins.

> Once food mixes with gastric juice and enters the small intestine it is called **chyme.**

Small intestine — a small-diameter tube connecting the stomach to the large intestine; longest part of the digestive tract (about 10 to 13 ft); where the digestion process is completed, followed by absorption of most nutrients.

> Small, finger-like projections **(villi)** on the mucosa of the small intestine greatly increase the available surface area for absorption.

  Duodenum — first 25 cm (about 10 in) of the small intestine; receives **bile** and **pancreatic juice** through ducts from the liver, gallbladder, and pancreas.

  Jejunum — the middle segment of the small intestine; about 6 to 8 ft in length.

  Ileum — last 8 to 12 ft of the small intestine; connects to the cecum of the large intestine via the **ileocecal valve.**

Large intestine — a large tube that connects the small intestine and the anus; absorbs water and electrolytes from the feces.

> Once food passes from the small intestine to the large intestine it is called **feces.**

  Cecum [*caecum = pouch*] — a large pouch that forms the first segment of the large intestine.

  Vermiform appendix [*appendix = attachment*] — projects from the posteromedial margin of the cecum.

  Ascending colon — ascends from the cecum along the right side of the abdomen.

> Although the **appendix** has no apparent function, it has been found to contain an abundance of lymphatic tissue, which would allow it to help resist or fight infection.

  Transverse colon — crosses the abdominal cavity from right to left just below the diaphragm.

  Descending colon — descends from the transverse colon down the abdomen on the left side.

  Sigmoid colon — an S-shaped section of the colon before the rectum.

Rectum — the last 20 cm (7.5 in) of the digestive tract.

  Anus [*anus = ring*] — last 2 to 3 cm of the rectum; provides the external opening; contains two sphincter muscles that control defecation (i.e., the process of expelling feces).

  Internal anal sphincter — a ring of smooth muscle.

  External anal sphincter — a ring of skeletal muscle.

Accessory Organs

Liver — the largest internal organ; made up of four lobes; highly vascular; positioned directly beneath the diaphragm in the upper right quadrant of the abdomen; functions include:

1. Storage of glycogen
2. Synthesis of blood proteins (e.g., albumin, globulins, clotting factors)
3. Destruction of old red blood cells
4. Manufacture of bile to break down fats (main digestive function)
5. Removal of toxic substances
6. Storage of vitamins and minerals
7. Synthesis of urea (waste product from protein metabolism)

Gallbladder — a muscular sac under the liver; functions as a storage pouch for bile (Figure 14–2).

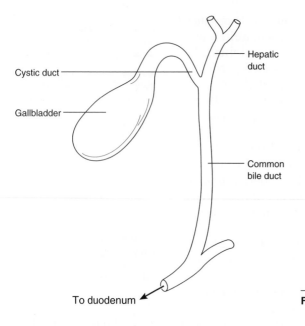

Cystic duct

Gallbladder

Hepatic duct

Common bile duct

To duodenum

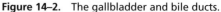

Figure 14–2. The gallbladder and bile ducts.

Pancreas — a soft organ positioned below the stomach and behind the peritoneum (retroperitoneal); produces an alkaline fluid called **pancreatic juice** that breaks down fats, proteins, carbohydrates, and nucleic acids (e.g., DNA).

> Because the gastric juice coming out of the stomach is so acidic, the alkaline **pancreatic juice** acts as a necessary neutralizer for the acid and brings the pH closer to neutral (pH of 7).

Bile ducts — tubes that carry bile from the liver and gallbladder to the duodenum (see Figure 14–2).

    Hepatic duct — carries bile from the liver; joins with the cystic duct.

    Cystic duct — carries bile from the gallbladder; joins with the hepatic duct.

    Common bile duct — takes bile from the cystic duct and hepatic duct into the duodenum.

Salivary glands — see *oral cavity*.

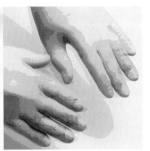

Chapter Fifteen

Urinary System

Organs of the Urinary System

Kidney — the main organ of the urinary system (Figure 15–1); located behind the peritoneum (retroperitoneal space) in the lower thoracic and upper lumbar region, against the posterior wall of the abdominal cavity; responsible for filtering the blood and producing urine; specific functions include:

1. Filtration of blood to remove wastes, excess salts, and toxins
2. Production of urine to excrete unwanted materials
3. Maintenance of water balance for the body
4. Regulation of acid-base balance
5. Production of hormones (i.e., erythropoietin, renin)

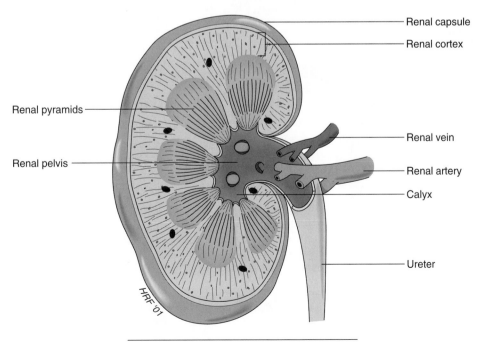

Figure 15–1. Interior view of the right kidney.

Hilus — the concave area on the medial aspect of the kidney; where the renal artery, renal vein, and ureter come into or out of the kidney.

Renal capsule — the outer layer of tissue surrounding the kidney; functions as a protective membrane to encapsulate the kidney.

Renal cortex — the outer zone of the kidney.

Renal medulla — the inner zone of the kidney; contains the renal pyramids.

Renal pyramids — triangular areas in the kidney that contain the nephrons; the apex of each renal pyramid contains many little openings (**papillae**) where the urine can drain out of the nephron.

Calyces (major and minor) — inlets on the renal pelvis that collect the urine from the renal pyramids.

Renal pelvis — an expansion of the ureter inside the kidney; collects the urine from the calyces and directs it down the ureters.

Nephron — the functional unit of the kidney; approximately 1 million per kidney (Figure 15–2).

Glomerulus — a network of capillaries where filtration of the blood takes place.

> The kidneys and the pancreas are **retroperitoneal,** meaning they are located behind the parietal peritoneum. This protects the body from any harmful wastes or enzymes that could be released when one of these organs is damaged.

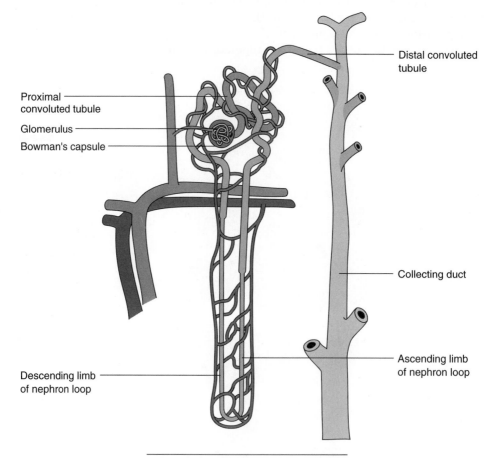

Figure 15–2. A nephron within a kidney.

Labels: Distal convoluted tubule, Proximal convoluted tubule, Glomerulus, Bowman's capsule, Collecting duct, Ascending limb of nephron loop, Descending limb of nephron loop

Glomerular (Bowman's) capsule — surrounds and encapsulates the glomerulus; receives the filtrate forced out of the glomerulus that will eventually become urine.

Proximal convoluted tubule — the first segment of the nephron tubule; reabsorbs about 65% of the water, reabsorbs many nutrients (i.e., glucose, amino acids, proteins, citric acid, ascorbic acid, calcium, potassium, sodium, phosphates, sulfates) and secretes substances such as histamine and some drugs into the *urine.*

Nephron loop (loop of Henle) — includes the descending and ascending limbs.

Descending limb — permeable to water only; absorbs about 15% of the reabsorbed water from the filtrate.

Ascending limb — permeable to salts (i.e., sodium and chloride) only; absorbs sodium and chloride from the filtrate.

Distal convoluted tubule — the last segment of the nephron before the collecting duct; reabsorbs sodium, potassium, and about 10% of the reabsorbed water when activated by antidiuretic hormone.

Collecting duct — the tubule that takes the filtrate from the distal convoluted tubule out through the papillae and into the minor calyces where it becomes urine; reabsorbs about 10% of the reabsorbed water when activated by antidiuretic hormone.

Ureters — long tubes that conduct urine from each kidney to the urinary bladder.

Urinary bladder — a holding pouch for urine located at the bottom of the pelvic cavity behind the symphysis pubis; lined with transitional epithelial tissue to allow for distension (stretching); has an average capacity of 700 to 800 mL (3.0 to 3.5 cups); contains a layer of smooth muscle to help expel urine during **micturition** (urination).

Urethra — a tube that transports urine out of the bladder; varies in length for males and females (male urethra = 20 cm or 8 in; female urethra = 4 cm or 1.5 in); also used in the male reproductive system to transport semen.

Internal urethral sphincter — involuntary smooth muscle; located around the neck of the bladder where the urethra emerges.

External urethral sphincter — voluntary skeletal muscle; located below the internal urethral sphincter.

Urine

Normal Constituents of Urine

Water (makes up nearly 95% of urine)
Nitrogenous wastes (e.g., urea, uric acid, creatine)

The **afferent arteriole** (blood vessel that brings blood into the glomerulus) is larger in diameter than the **efferent arteriole** (blood vessel that takes blood out of the glomerulus). This difference in size creates a mechanical pressure in the glomerulus that forces fluid and small particles through the pores of the glomerulus (**fenestrae**) and into the glomerular capsule. Because blood cells are too large, they do not pass through the fenestrae; therefore, blood cells are not normally found in the urine.

Remember that **antidiuretic hormone** is put out by the posterior pituitary gland in response to the body's need for water. It goes to the distal convoluted tubule and the collecting duct and stimulates them to reabsorb more water.

Because of the length difference between the male and female urethra, females are more likely to develop **urinary tract infections.** It is much easier for the bacteria to move up the shorter female urethra to infect the bladder. This results in the appearance of bacteria in the urine, which is normally sterile.

Because the urethra passes through the prostate gland in the male, **prostatitis** (inflammation of the prostate gland) can block the urethra and cause **urinary retention** (the inability to void urine). **Prostate cancer** can lead to a **prostatectomy** (removal of the prostate gland), which can disrupt the function of the internal and external urethral sphincters, resulting in **incontinence** (inability to control micturition).

Electrolytes (e.g., sodium, chloride, calcium, magnesium, potassium, sulfates, bicarbonate)

Yellow pigment (bilirubin, a product of red blood cell breakdown, from the blood is converted into a yellow pigment called **urobilinogen** that dissolves into the urine and gives it its characteristic color.)

Less than 1% of the volume of water that enters the nephron actually passes into the urine. This makes the urine about 65 times more concentrated than the filtrate as it comes out of the glomerulus.

Abnormal Constituents of Urine

Glucose
Red blood cells
Albumin
White blood cells
Ketones

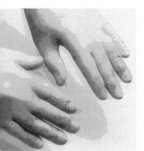

Chapter Sixteen

Reproductive System

General Terminology

Gametes — sex cells; sperm in the male and ova in the female.
Gonads — primary sex organs; produce the gametes.
    Testes — organs that produce **spermatozoa** (sperm) in the male.
    Ovaries — organs that produce **ova** (eggs) in the female.
Meiosis — the type of cell division in which the gametes are produced; daughter cells contain 23 chromosomes (half of the genetic material found in other cells of the body).

Male Reproductive System

Terminology

Erection — a process involving the accumulation of blood in the erectile tissue of the penis due to vasodilation of the arteries in the penis; causes the penis to become rigid and elongated.
Ejaculation — expulsion of semen from the ejaculatory ducts through the urethra.

Organs (Figure 16–1)

Penis — an external organ made up of three caverns of **erectile tissue** (two corpora cavernosa and one corpus spongiosum); contains the urethra; used to transport urine out of the body and to deliver semen into the female vagina during sexual intercourse.
    Glans penis — the distal portion of the penis; contains a high density of sensory nerve endings and serves as the area of highest sensitivity in the penis.
        Prepuce (foreskin) — skin covering the glans penis.
Scrotum — a sac located below the penis that contains the testes; contains a septum that compartmentalizes each testis; composed of connective and smooth muscle tissue (dartos muscle).

> The prepuce or foreskin is cut away in a procedure called **circumcision.**

    Dartos muscle — helps adjust the position of the testes to the body to keep the temperature of the testes about 2° to 4° lower than normal body temperature (the optimal temperature for **spermatogenesis,** or sperm production).

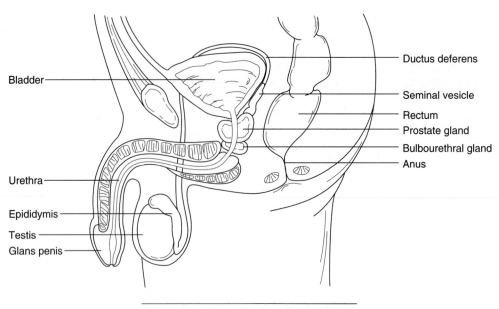

Figure 16–1. The male reproductive system.

Testes — the male reproductive glands; located in the cavity of the scrotum.

> **Seminiferous tubules** — the functional unit of the testis; long tubes in the testis that produce the sperm cells.

> **Epididymis** — a long, flattened tubule attached to the superior portion of the testis; functions as a holding area where sperm mature; also transports sperm to the ductus deferens.

> The seminiferous tubules produce more than 1000 sperm per second in a healthy, mature male. After the sperm cells are produced they must mature, a process that takes approximately 2 months.

Spermatic Ducts and Glands

Spermatic cord — a cord connected to the testes; made up of the ductus deferens, testicular blood vessels, nerves, cremaster muscle (helps the dartos muscle in the scrotum adjust the position of the testes in response to body temperature), and lymph vessels.

> **Ductus deferens (vas deferens)** — a ciliated tube that conducts sperm from the epididymis to the ejaculatory duct.

Seminal vesicles — glands located posterior and inferior to the urinary bladder; produce and secrete an alkaline fluid composed of sugar (fructose), prostaglandins (hormones that stimulate the contraction of the female reproductive organs to aid sperm motility), and other nutrients; makes up about 60% of the total volume of semen.

> **Ejaculatory duct** — a small duct formed after the union of the ductus deferens and the duct from the seminal vesicle; carries semen to the urethra.

Prostate gland — a walnut-shaped gland located directly below the urinary bladder; surrounds the proximal urethra, which is made up of smooth muscle that contracts to force the semen out during ejaculation; produces an alkaline fluid that makes up about 35% of the volume of semen.

Bulbourethral gland (Cowper's gland) — a pea-sized gland located beneath the prostate gland; produces a lubricating fluid that is released upon excitation of the male before ejaculation to clear out urine residue in the urethra and lubricate the tip of the penis; makes up about 3% of the volume of semen.

Urethra — a long tube that extends from the bladder to the tip of the penis; transports urine and semen out through the penis.

> Semen is made up mostly of water, electrolytes, nutrients, and hormones from the seminal vesicles, prostate gland, and bulbourethral gland. Only about 2% of semen is actually sperm. However, the sperm count of normal semen is approximately 50 to 250 million sperm per mL of semen.

Female Reproductive System

Terminology

Menstrual cycle — the reproductive cycle (about 28 days long) during which the uterine linings are developed in anticipation of fertilization; if fertilization does not occur, these linings are shed; controlled by four reproductive hormones: follicle-stimulating hormone (FSH), luteinizing hormone (LH), estrogen, and progesterone.

Organs (Figure 16–2)

Ovaries — the female gonads.

  Follicle — a small cavity in the ovary that stores the ovum (egg); stimulates the ovum to mature in response to certain hormones.

> Upon full maturation of the ovum the follicle bursts, releasing the ovum near the opening of the uterine tubes. This process is called **ovulation.**

Uterine tubes (fallopian tubes) — ciliated tubes that transport ova from the ovaries to the uterus; most common site for fertilization.

  Fimbriae — finger-like projections of the uterine tubes that surround the ovaries; sweep the ovum into the open end of the uterine tube.

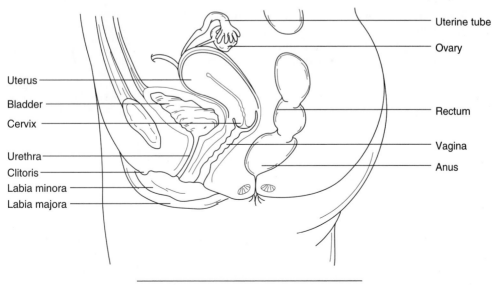

Figure 16–2. The female reproductive system.

Uterus [*uterus = womb*] — an organ shaped like an inverted pear; used for implantation of the fertilized ovum, growth of the embryo and fetus, and delivery of the baby.

Tissue layers

Perimetrium [*peri = around; metra = uterus*] — the outer serosal tissue surrounding the uterus.

Myometrium [*myo = muscle*] — the middle smooth muscle layer of the uterus.

Endometrium [*endo = within*] — the inner mucosal layers of the uterus; one of these layers, the stratum functionale, is shed every month and becomes menses.

Regions of the uterus

Fundus of the uterus — the bulge at the top of the uterus.

Cervix — the inferior portion of the uterus that protrudes down into the vagina.

Cervical canal — the opening in the cervix through which sperm travels to fertilize the egg and the baby moves during parturition.

Vagina — receives the erect penis during intercourse; functions as the pathway for the baby during childbirth; also called the birth canal.

Labia majora — the two large folds of skin covered with pubic hair that protect and contain the other external genitalia; composed mostly of adipose tissue.

Labia minora — the two small folds of tissue between the two labia majora that protect the vestibule; composed of nonkeratinized tissue that contains blood vessels and nerves.

Vestibule — the area between the two labia minora where the urethral and vaginal orifices are found.

Clitoris — the small, round organ found anterior to the urethral orifice; very high in sensory nerve endings; its only function is for sexual stimulation.

Breasts — the two lobes of adipose and glandular tissue positioned over the third through sixth ribs.

Mammary glands — modified sweat glands found in the breasts; produce and secrete breast milk.

Areola — the circular, pigmented region in the middle of the breast that surrounds the **nipple;** where the openings for the mammary glands are found.

> Implantation of the fertilized ovum usually takes place in the fundus or body of the uterus. Sometimes, however, implantation takes place in the uterine tubes or even in the peritoneum, resulting in an **ectopic pregnancy.**

> The acidity of the vagina functions as a protective barrier against pathogenic microorganisms but can be a harsh environment for sperm. This is why semen is alkaline—to neutralize the acidity of the vagina.

> During pregnancy and lactation, adipose tissue increases and mammary glands grow in the breasts, causing the breasts to increase in size. However, breast size varies considerably from person to person and is no indication of how well the mammary glands function.

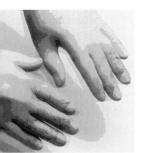

Chapter Seventeen

Craniosacral System

Significance

The influence of the cranium in health is an essential part of osteopathic medicine. It is believed that problems with the craniosacral system can affect a wide variety of health conditions. Many osteopathic techniques of manipulation and massage are used to treat these problems.

Involved Structures

Nerves — all of the nerves that control **parasympathetic** function of the body's organs originate from cranial nerves or sacral nerves.

Cerebrospinal fluid — clear liquid in the brain that supports or buoys the brain, cushions the central nervous system, and carries nutrients.

Ventricles of the brain — the four pockets or chambers in the brain where cerebrospinal fluid (CSF) is produced; the CSF circulates through the ventricles and into the subarachnoid space where it is absorbed by the venous system.

> Cerebrospinal fluid is produced at a rate of about 0.5 L/day (three times the total amount of fluid that is present at any time). Therefore, cerebrospinal fluid is constantly being absorbed as more is produced.

  Choroid plexus — the tissue in the ventricles that produces most of the cerebrospinal fluid.

Craniosacral Rhythm

History

The craniosacral mechanism was first observed in the early twentieth century by William Sutherland, DO. He theorized that the sutures of the skull are moveable joints, allowing the cranial bones to move. He also theorized that the beveled edge of the sphenoid bone, looking much like the gills of a fish, has a respiratory function. This led him to conclude that the brain expands and contracts rhythmically to move cerebrospinal fluid through the cranial vault, which he thought of as a type of respiration. Later, John Upledger, DO developed a modality founded on Dr. Sutherland's theory of a rhythm of cerebrospinal fluid movement in the dural membrane, but slightly different in approach.

Rhythm

Using the "pressurestat" model according to Dr. Upledger's theories, the production of cerebrospinal fluid is significantly faster than its resorption. Therefore, the rhythmic rise and fall of cerebrospinal fluid is achieved by some homeostatic regulation. Cerebrospinal fluid production reaches the upper threshold of pressure, then stops. The resorption, however, stays at a constant rate. This rate or rhythm generally stays at 6 to 8 beats per minute.

Palpation and Manipulation

Through gentle palpation and manipulation, the craniosacral system can be affected in a way that allows evaluation and treatment of the imbalances in the rhythm of cerebrospinal fluid production and resorption. This, in turn, promotes balance, amplitude, and symmetry of the rhythm that affects overall health.

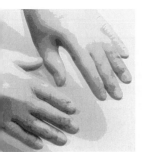

Chapter Eighteen

Biomechanics and Kinesiology

Body Mechanics and Safe Movement Patterns

Significance of Proper Body Mechanics

The use of techniques for proper body positioning reduces the possibility of fatigue and muscle strain. In addition, the use of proper body mechanics promotes efficient movement, which:

Increases strength and power
Increases pressure
Decreases possibility of injury
Enhances quality and effectiveness of massage
Promotes energy, or chi (see Chapter 20)
Increases career life span

Problems Associated With Poor Posture and Body Mechanics

Problems resulting from poor body mechanics are the number one reason why therapists quit massage therapy.

Wrists — overuse of the wrists can lead to problems such as carpal tunnel syndrome or osteoarthritis.
Back — poor posture of the spine and excessive leaning over can lead to neck and shoulder problems as well as muscle spasms and problems of the back and spine.
Arms — overuse of the arms can lead to nerve entrapment and fatigue in the arms and shoulders.

Postural Recommendations

Remember that the main source of strength comes from the lower body, not the arms and shoulders.
Balance on both feet with the knees bent.
Keep the back straight and head up.
Use the pelvis and torso to provide the leverage and strength needed to apply pressure.
Elbows and hands should stay close to the body.
Shoulders and wrists should stay relaxed.
Use substitutes (e.g., elbows, forearms, fists) when more pressure or relief is needed.

Tai Chi provides excellent methods for maintaining correct posture and body balance while performing massage.

Keep wrists and hands in alignment with the movement.
Avoid small, repetitive movements.
If injury or excessive stress occurs, rest until it heals.
Adjust the table height to allow for proper posture in relation
to client size.

> Do not work when you have
> an injury or illness, not just
> for your benefit but for your
> client's benefit too.

Proprioception

> Remember that massage
> therapists need bodywork on
> a regular basis too!

Proprioception — the special sense in the body that enables
us to detect body position and movement.
Proprioceptors — specialized nerve receptors found in joints,
tendons, and muscles that sense body position.
> **Muscle spindles** — proprioceptors mostly found in the
> bellies of muscles; provide information about the
> length or change in length of skeletal muscles.
> **Golgi tendon organs** — proprioceptors located where
> muscles join with tendons; prevent tendons from
> being torn by inhibiting excessive muscle tension on
> tendons.

> Damage to the central or
> peripheral nervous system
> (as in a stroke or peripheral
> neuropathy) or damage to a
> joint (as in a sprained ankle)
> creates impaired ability to
> sense body position.
> Therefore, people who have
> problems with proprioception
> have poor balance and poor
> coordination.

Lever Systems

First-class levers — allow variable mechanical advantage, depending on the lever arms
for resistance and force (Figure 18–1); also called "teeter-totter" levers; examples
include the ankle joint (plantar flexors with foot off the ground), atlanto-occipital
joint (extensors), and elbow (triceps).
Second-class levers — great for generating power but bad for generating speed (Figure
18–2); also called "nutcracker" levers; examples include the jaw (for back molars)
and the ankle joint (plantar flexors with foot on the ground).
Third-class levers — great for generating speed but poor for generating power (Figure
18–3); also called "baseball bat" levers; examples include the elbow (biceps), knee
(hamstrings and quadriceps), and hips (flexors and extensors).

Muscle Contraction

Muscle twitch — a single contraction followed by relaxation of the muscle.
Tetanus — a sustained contraction of a muscle; also called "muscle spasm."

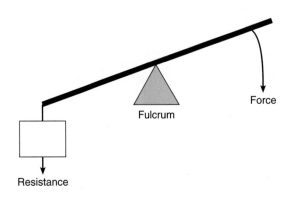

Figure 18–1. The first-class lever system.

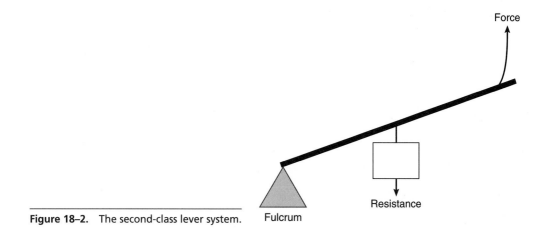

Figure 18–2. The second-class lever system.

Isometric contraction [*iso = same; metric = length*] — the muscle contracts but does not change length during the contraction.

Isotonic contraction [*iso = same; tonic = strength*] — the muscle contracts and changes length (shorter or longer) during the contraction; the same force of contraction is maintained throughout the movement.

> **Isometric** contractions are used to stabilize a body part to keep it from moving during an activity.
> **Concentric** contractions are used to accelerate a body part to produce a force.
> **Eccentric** contractions are used to slow a body part down or to resist a force after it has been produced.

  Concentric contraction — the muscle contracts and shortens.

  Eccentric contraction — the muscle contracts and lengthens.

Muscle Movement

Agonist (prime mover) — the muscle that is most responsible for a particular movement.

Synergist — a muscle that helps another muscle perform a movement.

Antagonist — a muscle that works against another muscle or performs the opposite movement

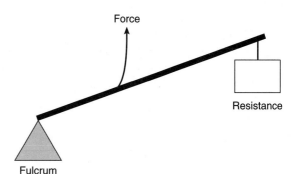

Figure 18–3. The third-class lever system.

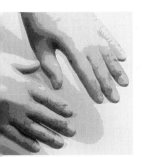

Chapter Nineteen

Medical Terminology

The Origin of Anatomical Names and Words

Latin and Greek Origins

Many anatomical structures carry their Latin or Greek name or a description of their size, shape, color, or function.

The Name of the Discoverer

Some anatomical structures are named after the person who first discovered them or discovered how they function. Presently, however, there is a trend away from using the name of the discoverer. In fact, body parts that bear someone's name are being renamed to reflect the position or function of the structure. For example, the bundle of His in the heart is now the atrioventricular bundle, the loop of Henle in the kidney is now the nephron loop, and the fallopian tubes are now the uterine tubes.

Commonly Used Terms and Word Roots

Because it would be impractical to provide a list of all the terms used in the medical field, Table 19–1 lists only the Latin and Greek word roots that are commonly used along with an example for each word root. Many of these word roots and their meanings appear in brackets next to medical terms throughout this book so that you can have a quick reminder. Remember that learning the meaning of the Latin and Greek word roots will not only help you remember the medical term itself, but will also help you learn or identify other terms that carry the same word root, prefix, or suffix.

Table 19-1. *Commonly Used Word Roots, Prefixes, and Suffixes*

Word Root/Prefix/Suffix	Meaning	Example
a-, an-	Without	Anesthesia
ad-	Toward	Adduct
adeno-	Gland	Adenoma
-algia	Pain	Myalgia
ambi-	Both	Ambidextrous
angio-	Vessel (blood or lymph)	Angiogram
ante-	Before	Antebrachium
anti-	Against	Antibiotic
arthro-	Joint	Arthritis
bi-	Two	Bilateral
brachio-	Arm	Antebrachium
brady-	Slow	Bradycardia
cardio-	Heart	Cardiac
caud-	Tail	Caudal
cephal-	Head	Cephalad
chondro-	Cartilage	Chondrocyte
cochlea	Shell	Cochlea
con-	Together	Conjoined
contra-	Against, opposite	Contralateral
crypto-	Hidden	Cryptorchism
cyano-	Blue	Cyanosis
derm-	Skin	Dermatitis
di-	Two	Digastric
dur-	Tough	Dura mater
dys-	Hard, painful	Dysuria
ecto-	Outside	Ectopic pregnancy
-ectomy	Surgical removal	Appendectomy
ede-	Swelling	Edema
epi-	Upon	Epidermis
ergo-	Work	Synergistic muscles, ergograph
ex-, exo-	Outside	Excrete, exocrine
for-	Opening	Foramen
gastro-	Belly, stomach	Gastric juice
-genic	Produce, create	Pathogenic
glosso-	Tongue	Glossitis
glyco-	Sugar	Glycolysis
hemi-	Half	Hemiplegia
hemo-	Blood	Hemolysis
hepa-	Liver	Hepatitis
histo-	Tissue	Histology
homo-	Same	Homosexual
hydro-	Water	Hydrocephaly
-iatric	Specialty	Geriatrics, pediatrics
ilio(a)-	Ilium	Iliac crest
infra-	Below	Infraspinatus
-ism	Condition	Hyperthyroidism
iso-	Same	Isometric
-itis	Inflammation	Arthritis
kine-	Movement	Kinesiology

(continued)

Table 19-1. *Commonly Used Word Roots, Prefixes, and Suffixes (Continued)*

Word Root/Prefix/Suffix	Meaning	Example
labio-	Lips	La bia majora
later-	Side	Lateral
leuko-	White	Leukocyte
lipo-	Fat	Lipolysis
lyso-	Break up	Glycolysis
macro-	Big	Macrophage
mal-	Bad	Malalignment
mater	Mother	Dura mater
medi-	Middle	Medial
mega-	Big	Splenomegaly
multi-	Many	Multiaxial
myo-	Muscle	Myofibril
neo-	New	Neonatal
nephro-	Kidney	Nephritis
neuro-	Nerve	Neurology
-ology	Study of	Neurology
-oma	Tumor	Neuroma
ora	Mouth	Oral cavity
orchi-	Testes	Orchitis
osteo-	Bone	Osteoma
oto-	Ear	Otoscope
para-	Beside, near	Parasternal
patho-	Disease	Pathology
-penia	Lack of	Thrombocytopenia
peri-	Around	Pericardium
-plegia	Paralysis	Hemiplegia
pneumo-	Breathing	Pneumothorax
pod-, ped-	Foot	Podiatrist, bipedal
-poiesis	Formation	Hemopoiesis
poly-	Many, much	Polyuria
pre-	Before	Premature
psycho-	Mind	Psychology
quadri-	Four	Quadriceps
rect-	Straighten	Rectus abdominis
reno-	Kidney	Renal
retro-	Behind	Retroperitoneal
semi-	Half	Semilunar
-sis	Process	Stenosis
somato-	Body	Psychosomatic
steno-	Narrowing	Stenosis
sub-	Under	Subdural hematoma
super-, supra-	Above	Supraspinatus
syn-	Together	Synapse, synergistic
tachy-	Fast	Tachycardia
thermo-	Heat	Hypothermia
thoraco-	Chest	Thoracic vertebrae
thrombo-	Clot	Thrombocyte
trans-	Across, over	Transverse
tri-	Three	Triceps

(continued)

Table 19-1. *Commonly Used Word Roots, Prefixes, and Suffixes (Continued)*

Word Root/Prefix/Suffix	Meaning	Example
-trophy	Growth	Hypertrophy
uni-	One	Unilateral
-uria, uro-	Urine	Dysuria
vaso-	Vessel	Vasoconstriction
viscero-	Organ	Viscerotropic

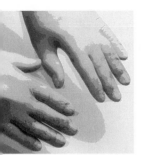

Chapter Twenty

Oriental Medicine

Five-Elements Theory

Following is a review of some of the main concepts of Oriental medicine to help you better understand this modality and how it relates to other modalities.

Chi — the "vital life force" that animates and gives life to the body; known as chi in China, ki in Japan, and prana and kundalini in Ayurvedic concepts; many other cultures also make reference to a life force.

Five elements — include fire, earth, metal, water, and wood; all forms of chi energy are interrelated and have one of these five elemental qualities; each element gives rise to another; everything is made up of one or more of these elements, but the human is made of all five, and when one element is out of balance the whole organism is affected; each meridian of the body has an elemental energy to perform the necessary functions in the body.

Yin and yang — the concept of opposing forces throughout the universe (e.g., light and dark, good and evil, positive and negative, male and female); founded on the principle that one gives rise to the other and cannot exist without the other; about a dynamic balance in all things.

Meridians

Meridians are energy pathways throughout the body in which chi flows to animate (give life to) the body and its respective parts. There are 12 paired meridians (primary meridians), with each pair having paths along both sides of the body in mirror-image fashion. In addition, there are the governing vessel and conception vessel meridians (extraordinary meridians) that circulate around the core of the torso. All of the meridians are connected to create one flow of energy. Yin energy flows from the earth up while yang energy flows from the sun down.

Primary Meridians

Table 20–1 lists the primary meridians in sequence to show the succession from each meridian to the next according to their position in the energy flow around the body. The meridian pairs share a yin/yang quality, beginning with stomach/spleen and continuing in pairs through lung/large intestine. Each pair of meridians starts where the last pair ends.

Table 20–1. *The Primary Meridians*

Meridian	Location	Element	Yin/Yang
Stomach (ST)	Starts at the eye, travels down the front side of the body, and ends at the second toe	Earth	Yang
Spleen (SP)	Starts at the big toe, travels up the medial side of the leg and the front of the body, and ends at the axilla	Earth	Yin
Heart (HT)	Starts at the axilla, travels up the inside of the arm, and ends at the little finger	Fire	Yin
Small intestine (SI)	Starts at the little finger, runs down the outside of the arm and up the neck, and ends just in front of the ear	Fire	Yang
Bladder (BL)	Starts at the eye, travels over the top of the head and down the back and leg, and ends at the little toe	Water	Yang
Kidney (K)	Starts at the bottom of the foot, travels up the medial side of the leg and torso, and ends at the chest	Water	Yin
Heart governor (HG) or circulation sex	Starts at the lateral chest, travels up the inside of the arm, and ends at the middle finger	Fire	Yin
Triple heater (TH) or triple warmer (TW)	Starts at the ring finger, travels up the back of the arm and the side of the neck, and ends at the side of the head	Fire	Yang
Gallbladder (GB)	Starts at the side of the head, travels down the side of the body, and ends at the fourth toe	Wood	Yang
Liver (Li or LV)	Starts at the big toe, travels up the inside of the leg, and ends at the front of the torso at the eighth rib	Wood	Yin
Lung (LU)	Starts at the chest and travels up the arm to the thumb	Metal	Yin
Large intestine (LI)	Starts at the index finger, travels up the arm and neck, and ends at the nose	Metal	Yang

The primary meridians are paired as follows: stomach/spleen, heart/small intestine, bladder/kidney, heart governor/triple heater, gallbladder/liver, lung/large intestine.

Extraordinary Meridians

The extraordinary meridians are not paired and are listed in Table 20–2.

Table 20–2. *The Extraordinary Meridians*

Meridian	Location	Element	Yin/Yang
Central or conception vessel (CV)	Starts at the perineum, flows up the midline of the torso, and ends at the lower lip	None	Yin
Governing vessel (GV)	Starts at the tail bone, flows up the midline of the back and over the head, and ends at the upper lip	None	Yang

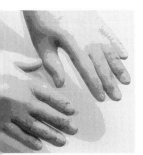

Chapter Twenty-One

Other Energy Systems

Ayurvedic Concepts

The basis of Ayurveda, or "The Art of Life," is thousands of years old, which may make it the oldest medical system known today. Those who practice Ayurvedic medicine and its concepts and philosophies believe that everything in the universe is energy manifested in many different forms.

No matter how solid an object may seem, it is still in motion at a molecular level; therefore, objects are always radiating energy and always have a specific vibration. With this in mind, everything affects every other thing, as energy is proven to interact. Human beings are energetic in nature and so are affected by the energies of the physical environment, nutritional intake, emotional involvement, and so on. We also affect everything with our energy, so we are all interrelating at an energetic level.

Ayurveda, like Oriental medicine, is based on the theory of the five elements (ether, air, water, fire, and earth). The five elements are the foundation of the body's ability to heal itself and define three doshas or tridosha (forces) in which the body intelligences act: Vata (air and ether), Pitta (fire and water), and Kapha (water and earth). Everyone is a combination of these forces, which together define our Prakruti (metabolic quality). Usually, each of us has a primary dosha that gives rise to our type of character. Vata types tend to be thin and energetic. Pitta types tend to be reactionary and short-tempered. Kapha types tend to be more subdued, slow to react, and solid. The idea is to keep these doshas balanced by using the entire environment to energetically influence our own energies. Ayurveda also holds that imbalances in the body are created energetically before the imbalance is manifested in the physical form.

Ayurvedic medicine uses different vibrational concepts in trying to alter irregular energy to a more natural vibration. This can be accomplished through the specific vibrations of color, environmental position, food, sound, and light. An example might be placing your bed with the head facing toward the east to take advantage of the energy of the earth's rotation, or eating yellow food to increase mental abilities.

The concept of vibrational medicine is crossing western barriers and, in fact, the oriental version of this concept (called Feng Shui) is turning architecture and lifestyle into an art form. Music therapy, light therapy, and color therapy are just a few of the many new types of vibrational medicine that are starting to be accepted as therapeutic, and are merely modern versions of an ancient medicinal practice.

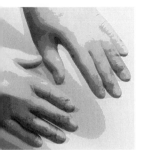

Practice Questions

Human Anatomy, Physiology, and Kinesiology

Multiple Choice Questions

Select the one lettered answer or completion that is best in each case.

1. The sutures in the skull are examples of what kind of joint?
  A. Synovial (diarthrosis)
  B. Cartilaginous (amphiarthrosis)
  C. Fibrous (synarthrosis)
  D. Condyloid

2. Which hormone goes to the collecting duct in the kidney to stimulate the retention of water by the body?
  A. Oxytocin
  B. Antidiuretic hormone
  C. Estrogen
  D. Calcitonin

3. Which of the following terms describes the relationship of the thumb to the humerus?
  A. Proximal
  B. Distal
  C. Internal
  D. Palmar

4. Which of the following muscles is MOST responsible for supporting body weight on crutches?
  A. Brachialis
  B. Triceps brachii
  C. Deltoid
  D. Trapezius

5. Which of the following represents poor body mechanics or poor positioning?
  A. Hands and arms close to the sides of the body
  B. Spine bent over to increase leverage
  C. Knees bent with weight balanced on both feet
  D. Shoulders and wrists relaxed

6. The rectus femoris, vastus medialis, vastus lateralis, and vastus intermedius together form the:
  A. shoulder girdle
  B. adductor muscle group
  C. quadriceps muscle group
  D. hamstring muscle group

7. The four muscles of mastication are the:
   A. masseter, temporalis, lateral pterygoid, and platysma
   B. medial pterygoid, lateral pterygoid, masseter, and omohyoid
   C. temporalis, sternohyoid, masseter, and medial pterygoid
   D. masseter, medial pterygoid, lateral pterygoid, and temporalis

8. The opening for the external ear canal is in which of the following bones?
   A. Frontal
   B. Occipital
   C. Temporal
   D. Parietal

9. What kind of bone makes up the main shaft of long bones and the outer layer of other bones?
   A. Compact bone
   B. Periosteal bone
   C. Spongy bone
   D. Sesamoid bone

10. Bones are attached to other bones by:
    A. periosteum
    B. osseous tissue
    C. ligaments
    D. tendons

11. The large bony prominence on the lateral aspect of the proximal thigh at the hip joint is the:
    A. lateral epicondyle of the femur
    B. greater trochanter
    C. ischial tuberosity
    D. lateral malleolus

12. The four muscles that form the rotator cuff of the shoulder are the:
    A. supraspinatus, teres minor, deltoid, and trapezius
    B. deltoid, pectoralis major, trapezius, and teres minor
    C. latissimus dorsi, tensor fasciae latae, sternocleidomastoid, and pectoralis major
    D. subscapularis, teres minor, infraspinatus, and supraspinatus

13. The blind spot in the eye is created because of the:
    A. optic disk
    B. conjunctiva
    C. fovea centralis
    D. retina

14. What type of muscle cell is NOT striated?
    A. Smooth (visceral)
    B. Cardiac
    C. Skeletal

15. Which of the following is NOT a purpose of the blood?
    A. Transportation
    B. Digestion
    C. Protection
    D. Regulation

16. The bile that is produced in the liver breaks down:
A. carbohydrates
B. fats
C. glucose
D. proteins

17. The pyloric sphincter is located:
A. at the end of the colon
B. between the esophagus and the stomach
C. between the stomach and the duodenum
D. between the small and large intestine

18. An isometric contraction occurs when:
A. the muscle contracts and develops tension but does not change length
B. the muscle contracts and shortens
C. the muscle contracts and lengthens
D. the muscle contracts and moves a bone

19. The ileocecal valve is located:
A. at the end of the transverse colon
B. at the end of the esophagus
C. near the common bile duct
D. between the small and large intestine

20. The pectoralis major, coracobrachialis, latissimus dorsi, and teres major all work together to cause what type of movement of the shoulder (glenohumeral) joint?
A. Extension
B. Abduction
C. Adduction
D. Flexion

21. Which class of lever is good for generating speed but poor for generating power?
A. First-class lever
B. Second-class lever
C. Third-class lever
D. Fourth-class lever

22. Urine passes from the kidney to the bladder through the:
A. ureter
B. urethra
C. urinal canal
D. urinoma

23. Where does the piriformis muscle originate and insert?
A. Originates on the anterior tibia; inserts on the first cuneiform and first metatarsal
B. Originates on the iliac crest; inserts on the lumbar vertebrae and twelfth rib
C. Originates on the pubis; inserts on the linea aspera
D. Originates on the anterior sacrum; inserts on the greater trochanter

24. The amount of air moved into or out of the lungs during quiet, relaxed breathing is called the:
A. tidal volume
B. vital capacity
C. residual volume
D. total lung capacity

25. Which of the following muscles does NOT help extend the shoulder joint?
A. Deltoid
B. Trapezius
C. Triceps brachii
D. Infraspinatus

26. A vaccination is a form of:
A. passive, naturally acquired immunity
B. active, artificially acquired immunity
C. inborn immunity
D. passive, artificially acquired immunity

27. Which of the following muscles does NOT attach to the os coxae?
A. Internal oblique
B. Sartorius
C. Vastus medialis
D. Semimembranosus

28. Which of the following is NOT a function of the lymphatic system?
A. Production and distribution of fat
B. Drainage of excess fluids from the tissue
C. Absorption of fats from the small intestine
D. Protection from foreign invaders

29. Type O Rh-positive blood has:
A. the A antigen, B antibody, and Rh antigen
B. the A and B antigens and the Rh antibody
C. the A and B antibodies and the Rh antigen
D. no antigens and the A, B, and Rh antibodies

30. Which of the following muscles inserts on the olecranon process?
A. Quadriceps femoris
B. Biceps brachii
C. Triceps brachii
D. Brachialis

31. Which of the following neurotransmitters is released in the neuromuscular junction?
A. Acetylcholine
B. Epinephrine
C. Norepinephrine
D. Dopamine

32. The central nervous system is made up of the:
A. cerebral cortex and medulla oblongata
B. 12 cranial nerves and the sympathetic chain
C. motor and sensory neurons
D. brain and spinal cord

33. The cranial nerve responsible for carrying general sensory impulses from the face is the:
A. trigeminal nerve
B. abducens nerve
C. vagus nerve
D. olfactory nerve

34. The spaces in the brain that contain cerebrospinal fluid are called:
A. centrioles
B. foramina
C. ventricles
D. pons

35. The portion of the peripheral nerves that helps prepare the body for the fight-or-flight response is known as the:
A. autonomic nervous system
B. neurotransmitters
C. sympathetic nervous system
D. cerebral sulcus

36. The visual center of the brain is located in the:
A. occipital lobe
B. frontal lobe
C. parietal lobe
D. temporal lobe

37. Which of the following is the proper sequence for the reflex arc?
A. Sensory organ, efferent neuron, interneuron, afferent neuron, effector organ
B. Afferent neuron, sensory organ, interneuron, effector organ, efferent neuron
C. Sensory organ, efferent neuron, afferent neuron, interneuron, effector organ
D. Sensory organ, afferent neuron, interneuron, efferent neuron, effector organ

38. Which valves in the heart produce the strong "lubb" sound?
A. Atrioventricular valves
B. Semilunar valves
C. Atrioventricular and semilunar valves closing together
D. Atrioventricular and semilunar valves opening together

39. The tympanic membrane divides the external ear from the middle ear.
A. True
B. False

40. Dendrites on the neuron receive information and the axon on the neuron transmits impulses away from the cell body.
A. True
B. False

41. The medulla oblongata in the brainstem contains which of the following centers?
A. Visual center
B. Cardiac center
C. Speech center
D. Motor center

42. The glomerular capsule is a vital part of which organ system?
A. Digestive
B. Urinary
C. Muscular
D. Respiratory

43. Which of the following regulate(s) the growth, development, and functioning of the reproductive systems in both males and females?
  A. Calcitonin
  B. Thyroid-stimulating hormone
  C. Follicle-stimulating hormone and luteinizing hormone
  D. Prolactin

44. What is the longest part of the digestive tract?
  A. Esophagus
  B. Stomach
  C. Large intestine
  D. Small intestine

45. What substance in the blood carries oxygen to other cells of the body?
  A. Hemoglobin
  B. Leukocytes
  C. Plasma
  D. Albumin

46. The outer layer of tissue surrounding the uterus is called the:
  A. endometrium
  B. myometrium
  C. perimetrium
  D. cervix

47. The interphalangeal joints of the hands and feet are examples of what kind of joint?
  A. Hinge
  B. Ball and socket
  C. Gliding
  D. Saddle

48. Which of the following is the proper sequence of blood through the heart?
  A. Right ventricle, pulmonary semilunar valve, pulmonary trunk, pulmonary arteries
  B. Superior vena cava, left atrium, tricuspid valve, left ventricle
  C. Bicuspid valve, aorta, lungs, pulmonary veins
  D. Right atrium, pulmonary semilunar valve, aorta, body

49. What is the sensory pattern on the skin for the axillary nerve?
  A. Over the deltoid muscle on the lateral aspect of the shoulder
  B. Palm of the hand
  C. Posterior forearm
  D. Fifth finger and medial half of fourth finger

50. Contractions in which there is no change in muscle length but a significant increase in muscle tension are known as:
  A. isotonic contractions
  B. isometric contractions
  C. concentric contractions
  D. eccentric contractions

51. Which of the following muscles flexes the neck?
  A. Latissimus dorsi
  B. External oblique
  C. Sternocleidomastoid
  D. Masseter

52. Skeletal muscle cells are also called:
A. muscle fibers
B. myosin filaments
C. myofibrils
D. myotomes

53. The lungs are located in the:
A. pericardial cavity
B. mediastinum
C. thoracic cavity
D. dorsal cavity

54. The rods in the eye see:
A. black and white
B. color
C. lines
D. motion

55. Where in the brain is body temperature regulated?
A. Hypothalamus
B. Frontal lobe
C. Cerebellum
D. Occipital lobe

56. Which of the following is the building-up phase of metabolism?
A. Anabolism
B. Catabolism
C. Homeostasis
D. Micturition

57. Lacteals are:
A. specialized muscle cells that produce adenosine triphosphate
B. specialized nerve endings found in and around joints
C. specialized ducts that carry hormones from one place to another
D. specialized lymphatic vessels in the intestines

58. What is an ion?
A. A positively or negatively charged particle
B. The product that results when an acid is added to a base
C. A substance that prevents sharp changes in pH
D. An atom that is at equilibrium

59. Which part of a muscle moves during a muscle contraction?
A. Tubercle
B. Insertion
C. Ligament
D. Origin

60. A bone fracture (break) in the hand might involve which of the following bones?
A. Scaphoid bone
B. Calcaneal bone
C. Radial bone
D. Cuboid bone

61. Which of the following is NOT part of the nephron unit?
    A. Proximal convoluted tubule
    B. Islets of Langerhans
    C. Bowman's capsule (glomerular capsule)
    D. Loop of Henle (nephron loop)

62. Which of the following is considered the pacemaker of the heart?
    A. Sinoatrial node
    B. Atrioventricular node
    C. Bundle of His
    D. Purkinje fibers

63. What are the meninges?
    A. Cartilaginous pads between the femur and tibia in the knee joint
    B. Membranous layers or coverings that surround and protect the central nervous system
    C. A group of glands that secrete regulatory hormones
    D. Tissue layers that line the organs of the abdominal cavity

64. Which of the following is a sympathetic hormone?
    A. Acetylcholine
    B. Epinephrine
    C. Adrenocorticotropic hormone
    D. Progesterone

65. Specialized nerve endings located where the muscle joins the tendon that function to protect the tendon from being overloaded are called:
    A. rods and cones
    B. Golgi tendon organs
    C. muscle spindles
    D. Schwann cells

66. Which gland is positioned above the kidney and secretes epinephrine?
    A. Pituitary gland
    B. Pancreas
    C. Adrenal gland
    D. Liver

67. What is the action of the minor and major rhomboid muscles?
    A. Protraction, upward rotation of scapula
    B. Protraction, downward rotation of scapula
    C. Retraction, upward rotation of scapula
    D. Retraction, downward rotation of scapula

68. Which of the following is the longest vein in the body?
    A. Great saphenous vein
    B. Jugular vein
    C. Brachial vein
    D. Basilic vein

69. The mitochondria:
    A. supervise cell division
    B. manufacture mucus
    C. produce adenosine triphosphate (ATP)
    D. provide cell motility

70. Which nerve roots make up the sciatic nerve?
   A. L2 through L4
   B. L2 through L5
   C. L4 through S3
   D. S1 through S4

71. The sagittal plane divides the body into:
   A. right and left sides
   B. top and bottom portions
   C. front and back portions
   D. internal and external portions

72. The ventral cavity contains the:
   A. cranial and abdominopelvic cavities
   B. abdominal and pelvic cavities
   C. cranial and spinal cavities
   D. abdominopelvic and thoracic cavities

73. Which meridian starts at the ring finger, travels up the back of the arm and across the side of the neck, and ends at the side of the head?
   A. Spleen
   B. Kidney
   C. Lung
   D. Triple heater

74. Serous membranes:
   A. line the inside of blood vessels
   B. are found in the organs of the digestive tract
   C. cover the central nervous system
   D. surround the internal organs and body cavities

75. What bones form the knee joint?
   A. Ilium and femur
   B. Femur and tibia
   C. Femur, tibia, and fibula
   D. Tibia and fibula

Matching Questions

Match the items in part A with the appropriate description or definition in part B.

Part A

_____ 1. Metatarsus
_____ 2. Sebaceous glands
_____ 3. Buffer
_____ 4. Anatomy
_____ 5. Myelin
_____ 6. Endometrium
_____ 7. Myocardium
_____ 8. Patella
_____ 9. Tachycardia
_____ 10. Orbicularis oris
_____ 11. Keratin
_____ 12. Humerus
_____ 13. Gonad
_____ 14. Occipital bone
_____ 15. Prolactin
_____ 16. Gallbladder
_____ 17. Meninges
_____ 18. Pons
_____ 19. Peristalsis
_____ 20. Axial skeleton
_____ 21. Cytoplasm
_____ 22. DNA
_____ 23. Olfactory nerve
_____ 24. Organ of Corti
_____ 25. Jejunum
_____ 26. Seminiferous tubules
_____ 27. Arteries
_____ 28. Bronchiole tubes
_____ 29. Acid
_____ 30. Ligament
_____ 31. Dorsal cavity
_____ 32. Pancreatic islets
(islets of Langerhans)

Part B

A. Bind bone to bone
B. Skull, vertebral column, sternum, and rib cage
C. Muscular sac below the liver used to store bile
D. Long bone of the upper arm
E. Cranial nerve containing sensory fibers for the sense of smell
F. Middle section of the small intestine
G. Fluid in the cell
H. Any substance that prevents a sharp change in pH
I. Kneecap
J. Endocrine cells in the pancreas that produce insulin and glucagon
K. Structures in the body that produce the gametes
L. Study of the structure of the body
M. Carries the genetic code
N. Carry blood away from the heart
O. Hydrogen ion (H^+) donor
P. Inner lining of the uterus
Q. Coverings of the brain
R. Hormone that stimulates the production of milk in the breast
S. Contains the receptors for hearing in the ear
T. "Kissing" muscle
U. Wave-like movement of the digestive tract
V. Bones in the feet
W. Lining around the neurons made up of neurilemma cells (Schwann cells)
X. Fast heart rate
Y. Oil-producing glands of the skin
Z. Cartilaginous tubes carrying gases through the respiratory system
AA. Part of the brainstem that has respiratory centers
BB. Muscular layer of the heart
CC. Contains the cranial and spinal cavities
DD. Bone that forms the posterior and inferior portions of the cranial cavity
EE. Protein that adds toughness to the skin
FF. Site of the production of sperm cells

Fill-in-the-Blank Questions
Muscle Origin and Insertion
Fill in the blanks with the correct muscle name, origin, or insertion.

Muscle	Origin	Insertion
1.	Zygomatic bone	Tissue in the corners of the mouth
2. Masseter		Ramus of the mandible
3. Temporalis		
4. Splenius capitis		Occipital bone; mastoid process
5. Sternocleido-mastoid		
6.	Upper eight or nine ribs	Anterior aspect of the medial border of the scapula
7. Pectoralis minor	Third, fourth, and fifth ribs	
8. Levator scapulae		
9.	Infraspinous fossa	Greater tubercle of the humerus
10. Coracobrachialis	Coracoid process of the scapula	
11. Biceps brachii		Radial tuberosity
12. Brachialis	Lower half of the anterolateral shaft of the humerus	
13.	Above the medial epicondyle of the humerus	Midlateral shaft of the radius
14. Brachioradialis		Styloid process of the radius
15.	Supraspinous fossa	
16. Teres major		
17. Latissimus dorsi	Thoracolumbar aponeurosis from T7 to the iliac crest	
18. Rectus abdominis		
19. External oblique		
20.	Posterior iliac crest	Twelfth rib; transverse processes of the lumbar vertebrae

Muscle	Origin	Insertion
21.	Lateral surface of the ilium	Greater trochanter of the femur
22. Piriformis		
23. Rectus femoris		
24. Vastus medialis		Tibial tuberosity via the patellar tendon
25. Psoas major		
26. Sartorius		Proximal medial shaft of the tibia
27. Adductor longus	Body of pubis; inferior ramus of pubis	
28. Pectineus		Between the lesser trochanter and the linea aspera on the femur
29. Gracilis		
30.	Ischial tuberosity; linea aspera	Head of the fibula
31. Gastrocnemius		
32. Soleus		
33.	Anterolateral shaft of the tibia	Base of the first metatarsal; first cuneiform
34.	Posterior tibia	First distal phalanx
35. Peroneus longus		

Review Activities

1. Trace the blood through the heart, including travel to and from the lungs. (Go through or pass by **13** structures.)
2. Trace a bite of food through the **14** structures of the digestive tract from the mouth to the anus.
3. List the **8** hip flexor muscles.
4. List the **7** shoulder extensor muscles.
5. List the **8** knee flexor muscles.
6. Identify the **5** lobes of the cerebrum and their individual functions.
7. Name all **11** of the organelles in the cell and describe the function of each.
8. Identify **6** facial bones by pointing to them on your face.
9. Identify the **3** formed elements in the blood and describe the function of each.
10. Trace the flow of filtrate through the **7** segments of the nephron and briefly describe what each segment does.
11. Follow the path a sperm cell follows from the seminiferous tubules out through the penis. (Include **5** structures.)
12. List the **6** hormones that come from the anterior pituitary gland.
13. Describe the **6** different kinds of synovial joints.
14. List **4** lymphoid organs.
15. List **15** nonspecific host defenses in the body.
16. Trace a breath of air through **9** structures of the respiratory tract from the nose down to the alveoli.
17. Follow a sound wave through the **7** structures of the ear from the auricle to the cochlear nerve.
18. Identify the **5** parts of the reflex arc.
19. Follow a red blood cell from the left ventricle to the top of the right foot. (Go through **8** different arteries.)
20. Name the **8** carpal bones and point to their approximate location in your hand or wrist.

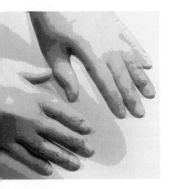

Part II
Clinical Pathology

Chapter Twenty-Two

History and Client Intake

Emotional State and Stress

Emotional State

A client's emotional state and the stress he feels both play an important role in his overall health. Feelings such as anger, depression, and sadness affect the body's physiologic processes in many ways and make an individual more susceptible to disease. (See Chapter 23 for a further discussion of emotions and their influence on disease.)

Stress

Dr. Hans Selye, a leading authority on stress, defines stress as "the nonspecific response of the body to any demand." All things require a certain amount of stress to function efficiently; it is when stress goes beyond elastic limits that it becomes "strain," or the structural loss of integrity. Dr. Selye concludes that most diseases can be related to some form of stress, such as can be seen when someone under stress has an increased susceptibility to viral infections. Following are 11 major categories of stress identified by Dr. Selye that can dramatically affect a person's state of health and well being:

1. Infection (overworks the immune system)
2. Injury (trauma)
3. Surgery (a precise injury)
4. Overexertion (e.g., overuse trauma, marathon)
5. Allergies (physical and emotional)
6. Immunologic reactions (e.g., drugs, inoculations)
7. Malnutrition (e.g., poor diet, lack of food, poor digestion)
8. Pregnancy (physical, hormonal, and emotional stress)
9. Strong emotion (e.g., death, divorce, wedding)
10. Exposure (extreme heat or cold)
11. Gravity (associated with body balance)

Past Medical History

As a clinician, it is important to be aware of the past medical history of your client so you can identify possible risk factors. Each of the diseases an individual has had, whether from abuse, trauma, exposure, or infection, can affect that individual's susceptibility to other diseases. For example, in the case of diabetes mellitus, circulatory and kidney problems, retinopathy, and infection can often result. A person who has more than one disease or condition may have more than two or three times the risk for other diseases because of interactions within and among the body systems. For example, a study conducted by Jick H, Dinan B, Herman R, Rothman KJ and published in *The Journal of the American Medical Association* has shown that the effects of smoking together with the use of oral contraceptives increases the chance of heart attack by eighteen times, a much higher risk than that presented by just smoking or using oral contraceptives alone (JAMA 1978; 240(23): 2548–52). (See Chapter 23 for information regarding other risk factors.)

Life Stages

Infancy (Birth to 3 Years)

During this time, a child is developing neurologically and physically, learning to sort through sensory information and to respond to it. As the child is exposed to new environments and objects, new health threats and sicknesses are presented. During infancy, a child's immune system is still developing, particularly right after birth, so the child relies on the inherited immunity that comes from the mother through breast-feeding. (See Chapter 32 for a description of passive naturally acquired immunity.) After weaning and through the early growing years, good nutrition, proper rest, and play are required for continued building of immunity and physical strength. Psychologic support and emotional stability are also of great importance during this stage, as good physical health goes hand in hand with good emotional health.

Childhood (3 Years to 18 Years)

During this stage, the child goes through great physical growth and development, including all of the changes that come with puberty. Growing pains, hyperactive sebaceous glands, and emotional swings usually occur and are the result of normal growth spurts and fluctuating hormone levels. Many of the common diseases of this life stage come from direct trauma (e.g., broken bones, sprained ligaments) or from direct contact (e.g., colds, flu, chickenpox). Psychologic problems often develop as individuals make the transition from childhood to adulthood.

Adulthood (19 Years to 60 Years)

During this stage, physical and psychologic maturation occurs. Many habits are developed, through demands at work or leisure time activities, that bear directly on the individual's health. Very few diseases are hallmarks of this life stage.

Elderly (60 Years to Death)

Many physical changes occur during this stage: muscle tissue decreases and is replaced by connective tissue, bones become more brittle, skin becomes thinner, and neither the circulatory system nor the nervous system works as efficiently as during earlier stages. With these normal changes come a host of new diseases ranging from Alzheimer's disease to varicose veins. Both physical and psychologic changes must be made to adjust to decreased functional abilities.

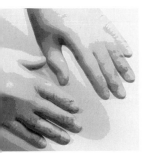

Chapter Twenty-Three

Introduction to Disease

General Terms

Disease — impairment of the health, condition, or normal functioning of the body.
Pathology — the study of disease.
Pathophysiology — the study of the physiologic processes of a disease.
Pathogenesis — the pattern of development of a disease.
Epidemiology — the study of the occurrence, transmission, and distribution of a disease.
Etiology — the study of the causes of a disease.
Mortality rate — the death rate for a specific region or population affected by a specific disease.
Morbidity — the ratio of those who are diseased to those who are well.
Endemic — disease affecting a community.
Epidemic — disease affecting an entire region.
Pandemic — disease affecting the entire world.
Diagnosis — identification of a specific disease or condition.
Prognosis — the expected outcome of a particular condition (including or not including different forms of treatment).
Acute — term used to describe a condition with an intense, sudden onset and short duration.
Chronic — term used to describe a condition with a less intense, long-term onset and long duration.
Local — confined to a specific area of the body.
Systemic — affecting the blood or the entire body.
Signs — outward, observable abnormalities (e.g., fever, rash, bleeding).
Symptoms — abnormalities that the patient complains of that cannot necessarily be detected by an observer (e.g., pain, fatigue, discomfort, achiness).
Syndrome — a certain group of signs and symptoms, usually with a common cause.

Etiology

Terms

Trauma — physical, chemical, or radioactive damage to the body.
Infection — invasion of a pathogenic microorganism.
Degeneration — the breakdown of body tissues, usually due to "wear and tear."
Autoimmunity — condition in which the body's own immune system creates an immune response to destroy its own tissues.

Risk Factors

Age

Each age group is susceptible to certain diseases that may or may not affect any of the other age groups. For example, premature infants are prone to respiratory problems, teens are prone to mononucleosis and venereal diseases, and the elderly are prone to bone fractures.

Gender

Some diseases may be limited to one gender, or at least more prevalent in one gender than the other. For example, males develop prostate cancer and are predisposed to hemophilia and muscular dystrophy. Females are predisposed to breast cancer, urinary tract infections, and lupus erythematosus.

Heredity and race

Some diseases are passed down genetically through generations so that different families or ethnic groups are more prone to certain diseases than other groups. For example, African Americans are eight times more likely to have sickle cell anemia than whites. Also, if a woman has a sister, mother, or daughter who develops breast cancer, her chance of developing breast cancer doubles.

Physical exposure

Exposure to the physical elements (e.g., cold, heat) can damage the body's systems. For example, prolonged or frequent exposure to the sun can lead to skin cancer.

Nutrition

Improper diets or diets deficient in certain necessary nutrients lead to disease. For example, a lack of iodine in the diet may lead to hypothyroidism or a goiter, and a lack of vitamin D may lead to osteomalacia (rickets). Diets high in cholesterol or fats predispose to atherosclerosis and coronary artery disease.

Congenital defects

Some diseases are present from birth. For example, cleft palate and spina bifida are both congenital defects.

Occupation

Different occupations predispose to certain diseases. For example, typists and massage therapists are predisposed to carpal tunnel syndrome.

Preexisting disease

Having one or more diseases can increase the risk of other diseases. For example, diabetics are more prone to developing kidney disease, retinal problems, and atherosclerosis.

Psychogenic influences

Mental and emotional health influence overall health. Factors such as anger, low self-esteem, hard-driving "type A" personality, anxiety, depression, and stressful life events all have been shown to be major factors in the development and progression of cancer and cardiovascular disease. (See Chapter 22 for a discussion of emotional states and stress.)

Life-style and habits

Certain life-styles and habits have been linked to disease. For example, smoking has been shown to be one of the most significant factors leading to lung cancer and heart disease.

Microorganisms

Virulence — the ability of an organism to cause a disease; a measure of the potency of a microorganism.

Aerobe — an organism that can live in the presence of oxygen.

Anaerobe — an organism that can live without oxygen.

Asepsis — the state of being without infection or contamination; sterile.

Disinfection — the process used to kill microorganisms but not necessarily bacterial spores.

Antisepsis — inhibiting microorganism growth; preventing microorganism reproduction.

Sterilization — the act of completely removing all living organisms, including bacterial spores.

Bacteria — small, single-celled organisms with no nucleus; found in virtually every environment; reproduce by dividing into two daughter cells (binary fission); come in many shapes and sizes.

>**Staphylococcus** and **Streptococcus** — common spherical bacteria; part of the normal flora (normal microorganism population) of the skin, nose, mouth, and mucous membranes; cause many different kinds of infections (e.g., "strep" throat, "staph" infections of the blood, pimples, impetigo, meningitis, bronchitis, pneumonia).

Viruses — single-celled organisms covered by a protein shell; not considered true living cells; have no independent metabolic processes; contain their own genetic material (DNA or RNA); when a virus enters a living cell, the viral genes are released and used by the host cell to produce more viruses; the production of viruses by the host cell eventually alters or destroys the cell itself.

Fungi — eukaryotic cells; multiply by budding and producing spores; grow in dark, damp places; examples include yeasts, molds, and mushrooms.

> Many **antibiotics** such as penicillin have been developed to fight against prokaryotic cells such as bacteria. Antibiotics will not destroy the cells of a person who has a viral or fungal infection because human cells are not prokaryotic. To fight against fungal or viral infections, an antifungal or antiviral medication must be used.

Inflammation

Phases of Inflammation (Table 23–1)

Signs of Inflammation

Redness
Swelling
Heat
Pain

Problems From Chronic Inflammation

Restricting range of motion — the presence of fluid around joints prevents normal range of motion.

> Inflammation can be either **acute** or **chronic**. Acute inflammation is brought on by a nonspecific injury, has a greater degree of blood vessel involvement, and usually subsides in a relatively short time. Chronic inflammation is brought on by persistent irritation and aggravation, is slower spreading, and leads to a larger amount of scar tissue buildup.

Table 23–1. *Phases of Inflammation*

Phase	Duration	Events
Initial phase	24–48 hours after initiation	Vasodilation
		Edema
		Some leukocytes attracted to the area
		Inflammatory chemicals released (histamine and serotonin released into surrounding tissues)
Migratory phase	Days 2–5	Start to see capillary budding into damaged tissues
		Epithelialization of skin
		Chemotaxis (inflammatory cells such as macrophages and lymphocytes attracted to the site of injury or infection)
		Inflammatory barrier established (macrophages and lymphocytes wall off infected or injured area; dead bacteria, macrophages, and lymphocytes accumulate to form pus or inflammatory exudate)
		Débridement or abscess formation*
Proliferative phase	Days 5–21	Repair cells called fibroblasts form scar tissue where normal tissue has been destroyed
		Cells grow in random directions and adhere to all adjacent tissues
Remodeling phase	> 21 days	Scar tissue reshaped and remodeled according to stresses on the tissue
		Cell pattern is more unidirectional
		Scar tissue cells are broken down and reabsorbed†

*Débridement occurs in superficial tissues; abscesses form in deeper tissues.
†Massage facilitates realignment of scar tissue and breakdown of unneeded tissue.

Adhesions — abnormal joining together of tissues surrounding organs and joints; may result from scar tissue buildup.

Excess scar tissue — scar tissue that accumulates due to chronic inflammation, replacing the normal active tissue; impairs the functioning of the organ.

Function of Histamine

Vasodilation
Increase blood vessel permeability

It is important for a massage therapist to remember that the purpose of massage is not to eliminate inflammation, specifically not acute inflammation. Each of the phases of inflammation (see Table 23–1) is the natural and necessary way the body heals damaged tissues. However, when inflammation becomes chronic, it becomes disruptive and damaging and needs to be stopped.

Allergic reactions involve the release of histamine from the tissues of the upper respiratory tract, which causes the characteristic congestion, running nose, and itchy eyes. Taking an **antihistamine** blocks the effects of histamine and therefore prevents these undesired reactions by the body.

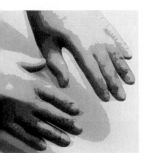

Chapter Twenty-Four

Diseases of the Integumentary System

General Terms

Skin lesion — general term for any abnormality of the skin.
   Macule — a flat, reddened patch of skin.
   Papule — a raised, reddened bump on the skin.
   Vesicle — a blister-like growth containing clear, serous fluid.
   Blister — a bubble of fluid below the skin.
   Pustule — a small blister filled with pus.
Dermatosis — any skin disorder, particularly one that does not involve inflammation.
Dermatitis — acute or chronic inflammation of the skin from any cause (e.g., sunburn, allergy, infection).
Pruritus — itching.

Tumors

Neoplasms [*neo = new; plasm = growth*] — tumors; abnormal tissue that grows more rapidly than normal.
Hyperplasia [*hyper = above, more than; plasis = formation*] — excessive formation of normal cells resulting in an abnormal number of cells.
Metastasis — the spread of a tumor from its site of origin to distant sites.
Benign tumors — nonspreading; localized; usually grow more slowly.
   Osteoma — a benign bone tumor.
   Lipoma — a benign fatty tumor.
   Nevus — a birthmark or mole.
   Papilloma — a benign growth on the skin or mucous membrane.
   Myoma — a benign muscle tumor.
   Angioma — a benign blood vessel tumor.
   Adenoma — a benign tumor of the glands.
   Chondroma — a benign cartilaginous tumor.
   Lymphoma — lymph tissue tumor (can be benign or malignant).
Malignant tumors (cancer) — able to metastasize.
   Mutation — a change or alteration in the genetic code.
   Sarcoma — a malignant tumor arising in tissue other than epithelial tissue.
   Carcinoma — a malignant tumor of epithelial tissue (i.e., skin, mucous membranes).
      Melanoma — a malignant tumor involving the melanocytes of the skin; represents about 2% of all skin cancers; greater than 50% mortality rate (most threatening form of skin cancer); may start out as a nevus that

enlarges, changes color, ulcerates, and bleeds easily; metastasizes very quickly.

Basal cell carcinoma — a malignant tumor caused by the development of neoplastic cells in the basal layers of the skin (stratum basale); accounts for over 60% of all skin cancers; appears first as a bump and then enlarges, crusts, and breaks open; hardly ever metastasizes to other areas of the body.

Squamous cell carcinoma — a malignant tumor caused by the development of neoplastic cells in the superficial layers of the skin (above the stratum basale); accounts for over 35% of all skin cancers; appears as a firm, red, keratinized tumor on the surface of the skin; can metastasize to the underlying layers of the skin.

> The main cause of skin cancer is exposure to direct sunlight. The ultraviolet (UV) light rays in sunlight penetrate into the skin, breaking down the connective tissue and producing mutations in the genetic code in skin cells. The American Cancer Society recommends using good sunscreen, protective clothing, and sunglasses to help block UV radiation and prevent skin cancer. Also, stay out of tanning booths! They deliver concentrated doses of up to 20 times the amount of UV light found in natural sunlight.

Bacterial Disorders

Cellulitis — noncontagious inflammation of the skin and deeper tissues.
  Cause: widespread bacterial infection (*Staphylococcus*).
  Contraindications/Indications: could be associated with a contagious condition; check with client's doctor.
Impetigo — a contagious bacterial infection of the skin; characterized by localized skin redness and vesicles around the nose, mouth, axilla, groin, hands, and feet that burst and form crusts.
  Cause: bacterial infection (*Streptococcus* or *Staphylococcus*).
  Contraindications/Indications: avoid affected area; check with client's doctor.
Folliculitis — contagious inflammation of a hair follicle; often contracted from hot tubs.
  Cause: bacterial infection (*Staphylococcus, Pseudomonas*).
  Contraindications/Indications: do not massage infected region; refer to doctor.
Acne — noncontagious inflammation of the sebaceous glands in the skin.
  Cause: hypersecretion of sebum (oil) due to hormonal changes in the body.
  Contraindications/Indications: do not massage affected area because it is sensitive and painful.

Viral Disorders

Fever blisters (herpes simplex) — open sores and vesicles around the lips and gums; contagious condition.
  Cause: herpes simplex virus type 1 infection.
  Contraindications/Indications: do not massage affected area.

> Herpes simplex virus type 1 is generally associated with infections of the upper half of the body while **herpes simplex virus type 2** generally affects the urinary tract and genital region and is therefore known as "genital herpes."

Chickenpox — a skin condition characterized by a rash that develops into pustules and vesicles lasting approximately 5 to 7 days.
  Cause: acute form of varicella-zoster virus infection transmitted through airborne route; grows in the respiratory tract and is spread through the body by the lymphatic and circulatory systems.
  Contraindications/Indications: do not massage; wait for rash to subside.
Shingles (herpes zoster) — an eruption of pustules along a dermatome (sensory area of skin innervated by one particular spinal nerve) of the nerve root.

Cause: delayed or recurrent form of varicella-zoster virus (VZV) infection; virus remains dormant in nerve tissue after a typical VZV infection that causes chickenpox, but may become reactivated years later.
  Contraindications/Indications: do not massage affected area; refer to doctor.
Warts (verrucae) — contagious infection of the epidermis; many different varieties (e.g., plantar, linear).
  Cause: viral infection.
  Contraindications/Indications: contagious; do not massage affected area.

Fungal Disorders

Tinea pedis (athlete's foot) — itchy, shallow lesions on the foot and between the toes.
  Cause: fungal infection of the feet.
  Contraindications/Indications: avoid affected area; refer to doctor.

> The term ringworm (**tinea corporis**) is often used to refer to a general fungal infection of the skin.

Tinea cruris (jock itch) — shallow lesions in the groin area.
  Cause: fungal infection of the groin.
  Contraindications/Indications: avoid affected area; refer to doctor.

Parasitic Disorders

Scabies — itchy eruptions that usually affect the webs of the hands, wrists, elbows, gluteal cleft, or nipples; papules and vesicles are very common.
  Cause: *Sarcoptes scabiei* (itch mite) infection.
  Contraindications/Indications: avoid affected area; refer to doctor.
Pediculosis ("crabs") — itchiness of the scalp, pubic area, or other places on the skin.
  Cause: blood-sucking lice transmitted through personal contact and sharing of combs, brushes, bedding, towels, and clothing.
  Contraindications/Indications: avoid direct contact with client; refer to doctor.

Other Skin Disorders

Psoriasis — chronic skin disorder characterized by oval, silvery, plaque-like scales with patches of red, especially on the scalp, ears, genitalia, and skin over bony prominences.
  Cause: unknown; suspected genetic influence.
  Contraindications/Indications: avoid affected area; refer to doctor.
Scleroderma (now called **progressive systemic sclerosis**) [*skleros = hard; derma = skin*] — an autoimmune disease characterized by deposition of collagen in the skin, lungs, heart, kidneys, and gastrointestinal tract; two to three times more frequent in females than males; most common signs include inflexible, cold-sensitive fingers and a "mask-like" face; can also experience esophageal dysfunction (difficulty swallowing or acid reflux), calcium deposits under the skin, and development of red spots, particularly under the tongue and in the mouth.
  Cause: autoimmune disorder; specific cause unknown.
  Contraindications/Indications: avoid affected region; refer to doctor.
Atopic eczema (atopic dermatitis) — noncontagious, general inflammation of the skin; characterized by blister-like formations that burst and form crusts; commonly involves the scalp, arms, trunk, and legs; may develop dry, pigmented areas of skin that begin around the elbows and knees and spread to the neck, hands, or feet.

Cause: unknown; may be an allergic reaction.

Contraindications/Indications: do not massage any areas that are painful, itchy, or weeping.

Lupus erythematosus — a chronic inflammatory disease that often shows periods of exacerbation and relapse; renal failure and central nervous system problems are most common causes of death, but can affect most body systems; 85% of cases are female; African Americans are three times more susceptible than whites; sometimes manifests itself as a butterfly rash across the nose and cheek, giving the appearance of a wolf (thus the name "lupus," meaning wolf).

Cause: autoimmune disorder of unknown cause in which the body produces an immune response against the nuclear components of the cell; suspected factors include stress, sunlight, and infections.

Contraindications/Indications: refer to doctor.

Urticaria (hives) — itchy skin eruptions.

Cause: usually allergic response to an allergen or irritating agent; may be influenced by psychogenic factors (e.g., stress).

Contraindications/Indications: do not massage any affected areas that are painful, itchy, or weeping.

Decubitus ulcers (bedsores) — dark patches or ulcerations of the skin that lead to necrosis of the skin.

Cause: prolonged pressure over bony prominences, usually from lying or sitting in one position for too long without moving.

Contraindications/Indications: do not massage affected area.

> Be careful of the types of lotions and creams you use. Some of the ingredients in these products can be the irritant that is causing an outbreak of hives. Try to use hypoallergenic products and ask all clients about any known allergies they may have.

Burns

Contraindications/Indications: check with client's doctor; avoid the area if painful.

First-degree burn — affects the epidermis; redness of the skin is usually followed by shedding of the skin.

Second-degree burn — affects the epidermis and dermis; redness and blistering; can leave scars when healed.

Third-degree burn — affects all layers of the skin and frequently some of the underlying tissue (e.g., muscle); open wounds with black charring and white patches of necrotic tissue; leaves scars when healed.

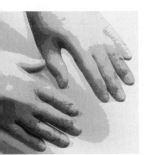

Chapter Twenty-Five

Diseases of the Skeletal System

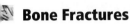

Bone Fractures

Contraindications/Indications: do not massage at the location of the fracture until there is complete union (usually 6 to 8 weeks from injury, depending on individual factors such as age); check with the client's doctor before treatment.

Simple (closed) fracture — a complete break in a bone without protrusion from the skin.

Compound (open) fracture — a complete break in a bone with protrusion of the bone from the skin.

Comminuted fracture — a bone broken into several pieces (shattered).

Greenstick fracture — an incomplete break in a bone.

Stress (fatigue) fracture — tiny, sometimes microscopic, fractures in the bone.

Impacted fracture — one end of broken bone is pushed into the other broken end of the bone.

Avulsion fracture — a piece of a bone is chipped or broken off.

Depressed fracture — a broken portion of a bone is pushed inward (e.g., skull fracture).

Spiral fracture — "twisting" fracture in which the fracture line wraps around the bone.

Nonunion — failure of the fractured ends of a bone to unite.

Malunion — faulty or poor union of the two fractured ends of a bone.

Skeletal Disorders

Kyphosis (hyperkyphosis) — exaggerated posterior curvature of the thoracic spine.
   Cause: spinal disorders (e.g., bone disease, poor posture, weakened ligaments) due to trauma.
   Contraindications/Indications: do not massage in severe cases; consult client's doctor.

Lordosis (hyperlordosis) — exaggerated anterior curvature of the lumbar spine.
   Cause: spinal disorders (e.g., bone disease, poor posture, weakened ligaments) due to trauma.
   Contraindications/Indications: do not massage in severe cases; consult client's doctor.

Scoliosis — lateral curvature of the spine; often creates a hanging arm length discrepancy and a "full chest" on the contralateral side; bracing is a common treatment; surgery is rare (only if very serious condition).
   Cause: leg length discrepancy, spina bifida, spinal nerve root damage.
   Contraindications/Indications: do not massage in severe cases; consult client's doctor.

Cleft palate — failure of the palatine processes of the maxillae bones in the face to fuse together during fetal development.

> A **cleft lip** or harelip (failure of the soft tissue over the lip to close together) may accompany a cleft palate.

Cause: nutritional deficiencies.

Contraindications/Indications: check with client's doctor; avoid the area if painful.

Osteoporosis [osteo = bone; porosis = porous] — loss of bone tissue leading to weak, fragile bones; commonly leads to postural changes of the spine and bone fractures in the pelvis, hips, wrists, and vertebrae.

Cause: unknown; influenced by hormonal imbalances and insufficient levels of vitamin D or calcium.

Contraindications/Indications: all bodywork should be light because although bones of the pelvis, lumbar, and cervical spine are most affected, all bones may be brittle; check with client's doctor.

Osteogenesis imperfecta — defective development of connective tissue, particularly bone tissue; bone tissue becomes thin and fragile and often bows under weight-bearing forces; often accompanied by multiple bone fractures.

Cause: genetic trait causing abnormal synthesis of collagen, an elastic protein that makes up about 90% of bone tissue.

Contraindications/Indications: massage is most often contraindicated; check with client's doctor.

Osteitis deformans (Paget disease) — common condition characterized by disorganized bone tissue reabsorption and reformation leading to thinning and thickening of bone tissue and overall brittle bones; microfractures are common; may be accompanied by deformed teeth, skull enlargement, osteoarthritis, nerve compression, and faulty hearing.

Cause: slow viral infection affecting osteoblasts and osteoclasts.

Contraindications/Indications: massage is contraindicated; check with client's doctor.

Osteomalacia (rickets in small children) — softening of bone and loss of bone mass; common in underdeveloped countries.

Cause: vitamin D deficiency.

Contraindications/Indications: massage is contraindicated due to the fragile condition of the bones.

Osteomyelitis — painful infection of bone tissue and bone marrow; sometimes pus-filled abscesses form; leads to necrosis and destruction of bone tissue.

Cause: staphylococcal or streptococcal infection resulting from bone fracture, surgery, or a penetrating wound.

Contraindications/Indications: massage is contraindicated; check with client's doctor.

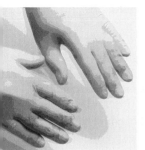

Chapter Twenty-Six

Diseases of the Joints (Articulations)

General Terms

Dislocation — displacement of a bone from its joint; usually involves damage to the surrounding tissue (e.g., ligaments, joint capsule, nerves).
   Cause: trauma.
   Contraindications/Indications: refer to doctor; do not try to reduce ("set") a dislocation; energy work is appropriate, but no stretching or massage should be done until pain and inflammation subside.
Subluxation — partial dislocation of a bone from its joint; sometimes referred to as "double-jointedness;" usually follows ligament injury.
   Cause: previous trauma; ligament injury; lax ligaments.
   Contraindications/Indications: use caution; energy work can be effective; may be advisable to check with client's doctor.

Disorders

Bursitis — inflammation of the fluid-filled pad between tendon and bone (i.e., the bursa).
   Cause: infection; trauma; overuse.
   Contraindications/Indications: avoid deep work on affected areas (in acute cases, massage can increase inflammation); use caution around all painful areas.
Tendonitis — inflammation of a tendon.
   Cause: infection; trauma; overuse.
   Contraindications/Indications: avoid any areas that have acute inflammation.
Osteoarthritis — most common degenerative joint disease; progressive, unsymmetrical deterioration and breakdown of articular cartilage, mainly in weight-bearing joints; loose bodies may develop in the joint space and react with the synovial membrane to cause pain; bone spurs may develop due to damage of the joint capsule; no known way of arresting osteoarthritis once it has had an effect; treatment includes weight loss, reduced activity, and replacement of the affected joint.
   Cause: "wear and tear" on the joint leads to death of chondrocytes and subsequent thinning and degeneration of articular cartilage.
   Contraindications/Indications: avoid areas of inflammation; be cautious of possible bone spurs.
Rheumatoid arthritis — severe form of chronic synovitis; stiffness and pain result from thickening synovium and projection of synovium into the joint; inflammation of the smaller joints of the hands, wrists, ankles, and feet is very common and symmetrical (affects both sides of the body equally); may also affect the heart,

lungs, and skin; signs include ulnar deviation of the fingers and radial deviation of the wrist.

Cause: autoimmune reaction, usually initiated by an infection.

Contraindications/Indications: avoid affected joints when in an acute and inflamed stage.

Gout — a metabolic disorder involving the development of tophi (masses of uric acid crystals with macrophages and scar tissue cells) in and around joints and the ear lobes; 75% of attacks involve the great toe, but other joints often become involved; affected joints are inflamed, red, and very tender; acute episodes can subside within 3 to 10 days.

Cause: 90% of cases are of unknown cause in which the body is not able to excrete enough urea in the urine; predisposing factors include alcohol and obesity.

Contraindications/Indications: avoid affected joints when in an acute and inflamed stage; refer to doctor.

Osgood-Schlatter disease — partial separation (avulsion) of the tibial tuberosity from the tibial shaft resulting in inflammation of the bone and connective tissue of the anterior knee; usually occurs in male children 10 to 16 years of age (i.e., during puberty); calcification of the tibial tuberosity is incomplete, making it more easily fractured; symptoms include pain when kneeling, running, climbing stairs, or riding a bicycle and disappear at approximately 18 years of age; usually necessitates bracing or at least decreased activity levels for an extended period of time.

Cause: "growth spurt" causing the bone to grow faster than the muscle and tendon.

Contraindications/Indications: avoid affected area.

Chondromalacia patellae — softening and deterioration of the articular cartilage on the posterior patella; pain usually experienced when forcefully extending the knee.

Cause: instability of the knee; substantial misalignment of the patella on the femur; overuse; chronic subluxation of the patella.

> Chondromalacia patellae causes significant pain, but in most cases the pain resolves spontaneously over time and does not necessarily progress to osteoarthritis of the knee.

Contraindications/Indications: get doctor's advice due to potential damage (particularly in acute cases); massage to and stretching of the quadriceps would be beneficial and could relieve the problem.

Temporomandibular joint dysfunction (TMD) — any kind of abnormal functioning of the temporomandibular joint.

Cause: trauma (often from motor vehicle accidents); poor posture; overuse from bruxism (teeth grinding).

Contraindications/Indications: TMD can change the position of the jaw, causing natural teeth, dentures, or bridges to fit together improperly; massage can relax muscles and relieve symptoms; work with dentist or physician if necessary.

Degenerative disk disease of the spine (osteoarthritis) — deterioration of the intervertebral disks in the spinal column; 80% of damage occurs in the posterior half of the disk; repetitive movements cause fissuring in the annulus fibrosis, which allows the nucleus pulposus to migrate into the fissure, reducing the potential for the annulus to heal; increased pressure in the outer annulus

> Some nuclear displacements are benign. Approximately 20% of people between 20 and 65 years of age have abnormal intervertebral disks but no pain.

may cause pain or paresthesia in the back or trunk (nerves are present in the outer third of annulus) or the pain may refer to the lower extremity; nuclear migration also leads to protrusion of the disk into the intervertebral foramen, which puts pressure on the nerve root, causing weakness and pain in the lower extremity.

Cause: poor posture; repetitive movements of the spine such as flexion combined with rotation when carrying or lifting heavy objects; low tension for long periods of time can cause the same amount of damage as high tension for short periods of time.

Contraindications/Indications: do not massage painful areas; check with client's doctor.

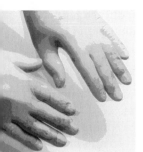

Chapter Twenty-Seven

Diseases of the Muscular System

 General Terms

Atrophy — a decrease in muscle cell size from either disease or disuse.

Hypertrophy — an increase in muscle cell size.

Myalgia — muscle pain.

> Remember that you cannot increase or decrease the number of muscle cells (or fat cells) in your body, but you can increase or decrease their size.

Disorders

Strain — occurs when a muscle or tendon is stretched beyond its elastic limits.
  Cause: trauma.
  Contraindications/Indications: use ice and energy work during the initial 48 to 72 hours; massage proximal to the injury may improve circulation and healing.

Sprain — occurs when a ligament or joint capsule becomes stretched beyond its elastic limits.
  Cause: trauma.
  Contraindications/Indications: use ice and energy work during the initial 48 to 72 hours; massage proximal to the injury may improve circulation and healing.

> **Strains** and **sprains** are graded according to their severity. Table 27–1 compares the degrees of severity.

Muscle spasm (cramp) — spontaneous, involuntary contraction of skeletal muscle.
  Cause: trauma; water or electrolyte imbalance causing the motor neurons to become hypersensitive and send out spontaneous action potentials.
  Contraindications/Indications: short effleurage from tendons to muscle belly can reset proprioceptors; compression, strain-counterstrain, proprioceptive neuromuscular facilitation, and reciprocal inhibition stretching techniques can be effective.

Table 27–1. *Degrees of Sprains and Strains*

Severity	Fibers	Swelling	Limitations
First degree	Stretched	Minimal	Minimal
Second degree	Partially torn	Moderate	Moderate
Third degree	Completely torn	Severe	Marked

Fibromyalgia — disorder characterized by abnormal patterns of sleep, diffuse pain and fatigue (particularly in muscles), headaches, irritable bowel, numbness and tingling in the extremities, and tender points.

> **Cause:** unknown; some suspect a genetic predisposition.
>
> **Contraindications/Indications:** use caution around tender points; kneading, pétrissage, and friction can break up adhesions and prevent further formation.

Chronic fatigue syndrome — disorder characterized by general fatigue.

> **Cause:** often associated with a chronic infection of the Epstein-Barr virus.
>
> **Contraindications/Indications:** massage may reduce associated stress and anxiety to allow the body to relax; avoid any deep tissue work that could overwork the immune system.

Torticollis (wryneck) — a deformity of the neck causing tilting or rotation to one side.

> **Cause:** spasm of the sternocleidomastoid muscle because of strain or infection.
>
> **Contraindications/Indications:** massage to neck (specifically the sternocleidomastoid muscle) will help relieve tension and anxiety.

Muscular dystrophy — a group of muscular disorders in which there is considerable muscle degeneration and weakness.

> **Cause:** inherited genetic trait.
>
> **Contraindications/Indications:** basic massage can relieve tension and related stress and anxiety, and could even slow atrophy; stretching can also be effective.

Duchenne muscular dystrophy — the most common form of muscular dystrophy; common signs, which usually appear before 3 years of age, include lordosis, muscle contractures, muscle wasting, and fat and connective tissue deposition in the muscles; patients are usually confined to a wheelchair by 12 years of age.

> **Cause:** inherited sex-linked trait (predominantly affects males).
>
> **Contraindications/Indications:** basic massage can relieve tension and related stress and anxiety, and could even slow atrophy; stretching can also be effective.

Myasthenia gravis — a disease characterized by destruction of acetylcholine receptor sites, producing overall muscle weakness; weakness is made worse by exercise and emotional stress and may lead to death if the respiratory muscles are affected; four times more common in women than men; incidence rate in the United States is about 3 per 100,000.

> **Cause:** autoimmune disease in which the body produces an immune response against the acetylcholine receptors in the neuromuscular junction; sometimes the cause is unknown.
>
> **Contraindications/Indications:** basic massage and range of motion exercises can relax and reduce stress; avoid any deep tissue work, which can release toxins in the body, stressing the kidneys and liver and potentially further complicating the condition.

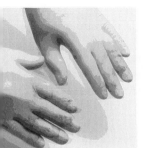

Chapter Twenty-Eight

Diseases of the Nervous System

General Terms

Neuralgia — nerve pain.
Neuritis — inflammation of a nerve.
Neuropathy — weakness in a distal area of a peripheral nerve as a result of trauma or degeneration.
Dementia — overall deficiency in memory storage, time and space orientation, language processing, problem solving and planning, and execution of voluntary movements.
Referred pain — pain felt in a region of the body distant from site of tissue damage or injury (e.g., angina pectoris).

Disorders

Hydrocephalus — increased cerebrospinal fluid (CSF) surrounding the brain; can accompany many other disorders.
　　Cause: oversecretion or impaired absorption of CSF; obstruction of CSF drainage pathways.
　　Contraindications/Indications: typically not a contraindication; may be prudent to contact the client's doctor before bodywork if in doubt.

Meningitis — inflammation of the meninges (coverings of the brain and spinal cord); 50% to 60% of cases are fatal if untreated, and 5% to 6% are fatal with treatment; infecting microorganisms invade the subarachnoid space and, together with cellular debris and fibrin, can block cerebrospinal fluid (CSF) drainage causing a rapid increase in intracranial pressure; leads to hearing and vision loss and brain damage; symptoms include fever, malaise, headache, lethargy, seizures, delirium, and coma.

> The term **meningoencephalitis** is used if an infection involves both the meninges and the brain.

　　Cause: bacterial or viral infection of the meninges spread from upper respiratory tract infection, otitis media, or pneumonia.
　　Contraindications/Indications: do not touch client because it is contagious; massage would be beneficial after medical treatment.

Encephalitis — inflammation of the brain; leads to nerve cell degeneration and ultimately brain damage; symptoms include fever, malaise, headache, lethargy, seizures, delirium, and coma.
　　Cause: almost always a viral infection transmitted through the bite of a mosquito, tick, or rabid animal or through respiratory channels.

Contraindications/Indications: massage is not indicated.

Seizures — sudden, involuntary, and sometimes violent contractions of a group of skeletal muscles accompanied by loss of consciousness.

Cause: increased electrical activity of the brain from injury, fever, or tumor.

Contraindications/Indications: massage is contraindicated during a seizure; deep tissue or painful massage is contraindicated for those who are prone to seizures; avoid perfumes or colognes (may trigger an episode); contact client's doctor if in doubt.

Stroke [cardiovascular accident (CVA)] — brain damage resulting from ischemia to an area of the brain; the third leading cause of death in the United States after heart disease and cancer.

Cause: blood vessel rupture or occlusion.

Contraindications/Indications: obtain the doctor's advice; generally, massage should be gentle and rhythmic; avoid pressure on any artery.

Poliomyelitis — inflammation of the gray matter of the spinal cord; sometimes results in partial paralysis (1% of cases); can be fatal if respiratory muscles are involved; other symptoms include those of respiratory and intestinal tract infections; antibodies are very effective in fighting poliovirus and the available oral vaccination should provide long-lasting immunity after one administration.

Cause: viral infection that destroys only certain motor nerve cells in the brain and spinal cord.

Contraindications/Indications: massage in postacute phase can increase circulation to affected areas, reduce anxiety, and promote muscle tonus.

Amyotrophic lateral sclerosis (Lou Gehrig's disease) — a disease characterized by loss of motor neurons in the spinal cord and lower cranial nerves; results in skeletal muscle weakness and eventual death; signs and symptoms include progressive muscle weakness usually beginning with the muscles of the mouth, throat, and extremities and ending with impairment of respiratory muscles; often affects those from 50 to 75 years of age; leads to death within 2 to 6 years after diagnosis; no treatment currently available; incidence is about 2 per 100,000.

Cause: unknown.

Contraindications/Indications: massage may sooth muscle spasm, improve motor function, and improve psychologic well-being; consult with client's doctor; involve a family member or friend in treatment.

Multiple sclerosis — a progressive disease involving demyelination of the neurons (plaques = areas of demyelination) in the central nervous system; faulty nerve conduction causes muscle weakness and uncoordinated muscle activity; affects people between 20 and 40 years of age; symptoms become worse and then resolve for a period of time, only to become worse again.

Cause: unknown.

Contraindications/Indications: caution must be used due to impaired neurologic sensitivity.

Huntington's disease — a progressive disease of the nervous system characterized by rapid, writhing contortions or rigidity of the muscles in the hands, arms, trunk, and face; leads to total incapacitation and death after about 15 years.

Cause: genetic defect affecting the frontal cortex of the brain.

Contraindications/Indications: massage may sooth muscular spasm, improve motor function, and improve psychologic well-being; consult with client's doctor; involve a family member or friend in treatment.

Spina bifida — failure of the vertebral arch (laminae and spinous processes) to close during early fetal development; condition remains asymptomatic unless the meninges or spinal cord protrudes.

Cause: genetic defect.

Contraindications/Indications: avoid the immediate area; general massage would be beneficial to reduce stress, muscle contractions, and muscle spasms; energy work would also be appropriate.

Thoracic outlet syndrome — compression of the brachial plexus or subclavian artery as it passes through the anterior and middle scalene muscles and under the clavicle and pectoralis minor muscle on its way into the axillary region.

Cause: tight scalene muscles; presence of an additional (or "cervical") rib.

Contraindications/Indications: use caution when working around the brachial plexus in the neck or axilla region (massage of cervical muscles, shoulder girdle, and pectoralis minor muscle could relieve compression and stress on the brachial plexus, but avoid prolonged, deep pressure in these areas, particularly if symptoms worsen).

Carpal tunnel syndrome (CTS) — most common neuropathy involving the median nerve in the wrist; symptoms include pain, paresthesia (tingling or partial feeling), anesthesia (numbness), or diminished sensation in the hand; common in people who work a lot with their hands (e.g., typists, artists, carpenters, massage therapists); leads to atrophy of the thumb muscles (often called "ape hand").

Cause: compression on median nerve from tenosynovitis (inflammation of the synovial sheath around the tendons); inflammation of the flexor retinaculum.

Contraindications/Indications: massage of the cervical muscles, pectoralis minor muscle, and muscles of the upper and lower arms are all indicated to relax the muscles involved and to improve circulation and nerve function.

Epilepsy — a condition characterized by long-term disturbances in the brain that lead to seizures; diagnosis depends on a history of at least two unexplained seizures.

Cause: increased electrical activity of the brain from unknown cause.

Contraindications/Indications: massage is contraindicated during a seizure; deep tissue or painful massage is contraindicated for those who are prone to seizures; avoid perfumes or colognes (may trigger an episode); contact client's doctor if in doubt.

Parkinson's disease — a slow, degenerative disorder that affects the motor neurons in the substantia nigra in the midbrain; flow of motor programs greatly impaired; symptoms include tremors (leading to body rigidity), bradykinesia (slow movement), tiredness, weakness, poor balance, mask-like expression of the face, slow speech, shuffling gait, and difficulty with fine motor movements (e.g., buttoning, handwriting).

Cause: loss of cells in the substantia nigra that produce dopamine (a neurotransmitter), resulting in decreased dopamine production.

Contraindications/Indications: consult with client's doctor; massage may reduce muscle spasms and associated stress and anxiety.

Alzheimer's disease — a progressive disease characterized by dementia and loss of memory (mainly short-term memory); the patient loses more long-term memory and suffers from personality fragmentation as the disease progresses.

Cause: genetic defect of chromosome 21, resulting in decreased production of acetylcholine (a neurotransmitter) in the brain.

Contraindications/Indications: massage can sooth muscular spasm, improve motor function, and improve psychologic well-being; it may be wise to include a family member in the client's treatment.

Sciatica — neuritis of the sciatic nerve.

Cause: trauma (e.g., falling); tight surrounding muscles; bacterial infection.

Contraindications/Indications: massage of the lumbar region and posterior thigh is usually very effective in reducing muscle spasm that may be compressing the nerve; if you see no improvement after several treatments, refer to doctor.

Bell's palsy — neuritis of the facial nerve (cranial nerve VII), causing paralysis of one side of the face; paralysis can be temporary.
    Cause: bacterial or viral infection; trauma to the nerve.
    Contraindications/Indications: overall massage can reduce anxiety related to this condition; use caution around the ear region.

Trigeminal neuralgia (tic douloureux) — degeneration or compression of the trigeminal nerve with associated neuralgia or pain along the nerve distribution.
    Cause: trauma; compression of nerve.
    Contraindications/Indications: avoid the entire facial region as massage may aggravate the condition.

Cerebral palsy — collection of permanent, nonprogressive motor disabilities; lesions affect certain motor areas and sometimes other areas of the brain, resulting in impairment of motor movement (spastic paralysis) or mental impairment.
    Cause: derived from perinatal brain injury (e.g., trauma, infection, toxemia).
    Contraindications/Indications: check with the client's doctor; avoid any deep tissue work.

Headache — pain felt in the head or upper neck.
    Tension headache — most common form of headache; compression of blood vessels and nerves occurs because of sustained contraction of the muscles of the neck and scalp.
        Cause: stress; overuse; sustained, awkward positioning of the neck.
        Contraindications/Indications: massage to posterior head, neck, and shoulders is very effective in relaxing tense muscles.
    Migraine (vascular headache) — vasoconstriction followed by vasodilation of cerebral blood vessels; characterized by intense throbbing pain, flashing lights, blind spots, double vision, nausea, light sensitivity, and hallucinations.
        Cause: stress; caffeine; oral contraceptives; cigarette smoke; various foods and smells.
        Contraindications/Indications: massage of the neck and shoulders may be very beneficial; use caution during an acute episode; check with doctor if necessary.

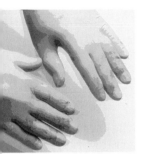

Chapter Twenty-Nine

Diseases of the Sensory System

Diseases of the Eye

Astigmatism — abnormal refraction of light coming into the eye.
    Cause: irregular curvature of the cornea or lens of unknown cause.
    Contraindications/Indications: none.
Myopia — nearsightedness.
    Cause: elongation of the eyeball causing the image to focus too far forward, before it reaches the retina.
    Contraindications/Indications: none.
Hyperopia — farsightedness.
    Cause: compaction of the eyeball causing the image to focus behind the retina.
    Contraindications/Indications: none.
Nyctalopia — night blindness.
    Cause: retinal degeneration; vitamin A deficiency.
    Contraindications/Indications: none.
Presbyopia — farsightedness in older adults.
    Cause: advancing age.
    Contraindications/Indications: none.
Conjunctivitis (pinkeye) — inflammation of the conjunctiva.
    Cause: bacterial or viral infection; allergies; trauma.
    Contraindications/Indications: highly contagious; refer to doctor before performing bodywork.
Strabismus — deviation of the eyes.
    Convergent strabismus — medial deviation of one eye.
    Divergent strabismus — lateral deviation of one eye.
    Causes: inherited trait; trauma or injury to the eye or the brain.
    Contraindications/Indications: none.
Glaucoma — a condition in which excessive pressure builds up within the eye.
    Causes: obstruction (usually of hereditary origin) of the outflow of aqueous humor from the eye due to a blockage in the canal of Schlemm (the canal that drains the aqueous humor from the anterior chamber).
    Contraindications/Indications: facial massage can reduce the stress from eyestrain.
Cataract — clouding of the lens or cornea that blocks light rays from entering the eye.
    Cause: trauma; exposure to the elements; degeneration due to advancing age.
    Contraindications/Indications: none.

Diseases of the Ear

Presbycusis — progressive loss of hearing in older adults.
> **Cause:** advancing age.
> **Contraindications/Indications:** none.

Tinnitus — ringing in the ear.
> **Cause:** presbyacusis; ear infections; otosclerosis; head injury.
> **Contraindications/Indications:** use caution when working around the ears; massage in this area may loosen fluid buildup in the inner ear; craniosacral work may be effective.

Otitis media — inflammation of the middle ear; common in young children; painful condition leading to fever and diminished hearing.
> **Cause:** microbes spread from an upper respiratory infection through the internal auditory canal (eustachian tube) and infect the middle ear.
> **Contraindications/Indications:** refer to doctor before performing any bodywork.

Otitis interna (labyrinthitis) — inflammation of the internal ear; usually produces vertigo (dizziness), loss of balance, and nausea.
> **Cause:** microbial infection of the inner ear.
> **Contraindications/Indications:** refer to doctor before performing any bodywork.

Ménière disease — a disorder involving the labyrinth of the inner ear; usually lasts for a few years; leads to a progressive loss of hearing in the affected ear, accompanied by attacks of dizziness, nausea, vomiting, sensitivity to loud sounds, tinnitus, and headache that can last for minutes or hours; most common among men between 40 and 60 years of age.
> **Cause:** most cases are of unknown cause; head injury; middle ear infection.
> **Contraindications/Indications:** for acute situations, bed rest is the treatment of choice; overall massage for relaxation can be effective; craniosacral work may also be effective.

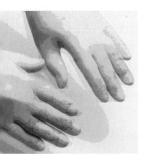

Chapter Thirty

Diseases of the Endocrine System

Acromegaly — hypersecretion of growth hormone in adults; characterized by hyperglycemia, thickened, coarse skin, and enlargement of the head, jaw, nose, tongue, ears, hands, feet, and some internal organs.
Cause: usually caused by an adenoma of the anterior pituitary gland.
Contraindications/Indications: none.

Gigantism — rare hypersecretion of growth hormone during childhood; leads to increased bone thickness and length and increased soft tissue thickness; accompanied by hyperglycemia.
Cause: usually caused by an adenoma of the anterior pituitary gland.
Contraindications/Indications: none

Dwarfism — deficiency of growth hormone during childhood; leads to decreased bone growth, short stature, hypoglycemia, muscle weakness, and retarded sexual development.
Cause: disturbances or trauma to the hypothalamus or anterior pituitary gland.
Contraindications/Indications: none.

Diabetes insipidus — a disease characterized by a deficiency of antidiuretic hormone (ADH) from the posterior pituitary gland.
Cause: inflammation or trauma to the hypothalamus or posterior pituitary gland; radiation to the hypothalamus.
Contraindications/Indications: refer to doctor.

Graves' disease — hypersecretion of thyroid hormones (hyperthyroidism); affects eight to ten times more women than men, usually between 30 and 50 years of age; leads to increased basal metabolic rate, weight loss, nervousness, fatigue, insomnia, diarrhea, heat sensitivity, increased sweating, tachycardia, and exophthalmos (protrusion of the eyeballs).
Cause: autoimmune disorder producing antibodies that bind to the thyroid-stimulating hormone (TSH) receptor sites and mimic the action of TSH, causing an increase in production of thyroid hormones.
Contraindications/Indications: refer to doctor; massage is indicated and beneficial if no infection, inflammation, or tumor is present; avoid anterior portion of the neck.

Myxedema — hyposecretion of thyroid hormones in adults (hypothyroidism); characterized by fatigue, slowing of physical and mental activity, swelling around the eyes, cold intolerance, and coarsening of the skin, particularly on the face.
Cause: damaged thyroid gland; hereditary defects.
Contraindications/Indications: refer to doctor; massage is indicated if no infection, inflammation, or tumor is present; avoid anterior portion of the neck.

Cretinism — hyposecretion of thyroid hormones in children (hypothyroidism); similar characteristics to myxedema, including swelling around the eyes, coarsening of the skin, and, depending on the age of onset, variable amounts of retarded bone and brain development.
Cause: damaged thyroid gland; hereditary defects.
Contraindications/Indications: refer to doctor; massage is indicated if no infection, inflammation, or tumor is present; avoid anterior portion of the neck.
Goiter — enlargement of the thyroid gland.
Cause: iodine deficiency (↓ iodine → ↓ thyroid hormones → ↑ thyroid-stimulating hormone → ↑ thyroid growth).
Contraindications/Indications: refer to doctor.
Diabetes mellitus — a group of disorders involving the pancreas; characterized by defective insulin response and/or utilization.

Insulin-dependent diabetes mellitus (IDDM) [juvenile-onset diabetes; type 1 diabetes mellitus] — characterized by a deficiency of insulin production by the pancreas resulting from a reduction in beta cells in the pancreatic islet cells; onset is usually before the age of 20; accounts for 10% to 20% of total cases of diabetes; hyperglycemia and polyuria (increased urine production) are common signs; treated with daily insulin injections.
Cause: genetic susceptibility along with autoimmunity to beta cells.
Contraindications/Indications: obtain doctor's approval and advice.

Non-insulin-dependent diabetes mellitus (NIDDM) [adult-onset diabetes; type 2 diabetes mellitus] — often seen in obese patients over 40 years of age; accounts for most cases of diabetes; treated with exercise and diet therapy.
Cause: insulin resistance based on decreased receptor sensitivity on target tissues in the body; reduction in insulin production.
Contraindications/Indications: obtain doctor's approval and advice.

Cushing's disease — a disease characterized by excessive production of cortisol from the adrenal cortex; leads to obesity, weakness, fatigue, menstrual abnormalities, hypertension, and a rounded "moon face."
Cause: hypersecretion of adrenocorticotropic hormone from the anterior pituitary gland; cortisol-secreting tumor.
Contraindications/Indications: due to possible complications (e.g., osteoporosis), all massage should be light and relaxing; energy techniques may be most effective; contact the doctor before performing bodywork if in doubt.
Addison's disease — destruction of the adrenal glands leading to decreased production of adrenal hormones;

The chemical **iodine** is used as the backbone for making thyroid hormones. Without sufficient amounts of dietary iodine, the body is not able to produce the proper amounts of thyroid hormones.

Both types of **diabetes** are accompanied by many serious complications, including myocardial infarction, ketoacidosis (decreased pH of the blood due to abnormally high ketones), stroke, peripheral neuropathy, decreased wound healing, gangrene (particularly in the lower extremities), retinopathy (leading to blindness), kidney problems, and increased susceptibility to infection.

As of July 1997, the American Diabetes Association changed "type I" and "type II" diabetes to "type 1" and "type 2" diabetes.

In Addison's disease, the production of adrenal hormones decreases dramatically, causing an increase in adrenocortico-tropic hormone (ACTH) production from the anterior pituitary gland. This ACTH is broken down in the body; one of the byproducts is **melanocyte-stimulating hormone (MSH).** This hormone activates the melanocytes in the skin to cause the characteristic "bronzing" of the skin for those with Addison's disease.

results in muscle weakness, fatigue, hypotension, nausea, decreased tolerance for stress, and "bronzing" of the skin due to increased production of adrenocorticotropic hormone.

Cause: autoimmunity against the adrenal gland; bacterial or viral infection; cancer.
Contraindications/Indications: refer to doctor.

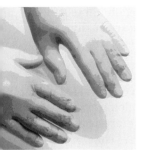

Chapter Thirty-One

Diseases of the Cardiovascular System

General Terms

Hypoxia — deficiency of oxygen.
Anoxia — absence of oxygen.
Ischemia — a lack of blood supply; results in decreased oxygen and nutrient supply.
Necrosis — cell or tissue death.
  Gangrene — necrotic tissue that has become invaded with anaerobic microorganisms.
Thrombus — a stationary blood clot in a blood vessel.
Embolus — a free-floating blood clot, clump of fat, mass of cholesterol crystals, mass of tissue, or even a mass of bacteria.
Cyanosis — bluish discoloration of the skin caused by a deficiency of oxygen in the blood.

> The most common clinical term used to describe the presence of blood clots in vessels is **deep venous thrombosis (DVT).** Massage is contraindicated for a client that is diagnosed with DVT.

Disorders

Hypertension — high blood pressure ($\geq$ 140 mm Hg for systolic pressure and $\geq$ 90 mm Hg for diastolic pressure).
  Cause: exact cause is unknown, but many factors contribute (e.g., old age, obesity, smoking, genetic factors, stress).
  Contraindications/Indications: check with client's doctor.
Hypotension — low blood pressure (< 100 mm Hg for systolic pressure).
  Cause: overall good health; blood loss.
  Contraindications/Indications: check with client's doctor; be careful when the client sits up or stands after massage is completed.
Anemia — a decrease in the oxygen-carrying capacity of the blood; accompanied by dizziness, fatigue, nausea, lightheadedness, and pale coloration of the skin.
  Cause: see following definitions of specific types of anemia.
  Contraindications/Indications: avoid massage because extreme fluid movement or pressure on the surface vessels may be harmful.

> **Hypertension** is considered a dangerous health risk. Those with hypertension are more likely to develop cardiovascular disease and have a decreased life expectancy. **Hypotension,** on the other hand, is usually no cause for concern. Those with hypotension have a longer life expectancy and fewer diseases in old age.

Sickle cell anemia — a genetic condition causing malformed hemoglobin molecules; produces fragile sickle- or crescent-shaped red blood cells that are easily destroyed; causes thickening of the blood, which strains the heart and reduces blood flow.

Hemorrhagic anemia — anemia resulting from a loss of blood volume.

Hemolytic anemia — anemia resulting from excessive destruction of red blood cells.

Iron deficiency anemia — anemia resulting from decreased hemoglobin production (and therefore red blood cell formation); caused by a lack of dietary iron.

Aplastic anemia — anemia in which the number of functioning stem cells in the bone marrow is decreased; results from drugs, chemicals, radiation, or cancer.

Pernicious anemia — anemia resulting from deficiency or malabsorption of vitamin B_{12}.

Leukemia — a disease in which many immature and ineffective white blood cells (WBCs) are produced; classified according to the type of predominant WBC, the severity of symptoms, and the total WBC count.

Cause: genetic disease in which malignant stem cells develop in the bone marrow.

Contraindications/Indications: obtain doctor's approval before doing any bodywork; all massage should be light because of the tendency for bleeding and bruising; energy work could be beneficial.

Hemophilia — a disorder characterized by the inability to form a blood clot because of a deficiency of blood clotting factors (e.g., classic hemophilia is caused by a deficiency of clotting factor VII).

Cause: sex-linked genetic disorder.

Contraindications/Indications: seek advice of client's doctor; massage should be very light so as not to cause tissue damage or bruising; use universal precautions in case of bleeding; energy work can be beneficial.

> Keep in mind that with **hemophilia,** the problem lies in deficiency of a clotting factor, not deficiency of platelets. In hemophiliacs, a normal platelet plug forms, but the bleeding resumes hours later because no fibrin clot has formed.

Shock — a condition in which there is inadequate delivery of oxygenated blood to the tissues, particularly to the central nervous system; signs and symptoms include pale or bluish skin, overall weakness, rapid and faint pulse, restless and anxious behavior, severe thirst, nausea, dilated pupils, sweating, and shallow and rapid breathing.

Cause: see following definitions of specific types of shock.

Contraindications/Indications: massage is contraindicated; refer to first aid procedures.

Hypovolemic shock — shock caused by a decrease in blood volume because of hemorrhage or excessive fluid loss.

Cardiogenic shock — shock caused by inadequate pumping action of the heart; usually the result of myocardial infarction; leads to decreased blood pressure.

Septic shock — shock caused by bacterial infection; results in localized vasodilation and increased blood vessel permeability, and thus decreased blood pressure.

Anaphylactic shock — shock caused by systemic release of a large amount of histamine during an allergic response; results in widespread vasodilation and increased blood vessel permeability, and thus decreased blood pressure.

Arrhythmia — an abnormal or irregular heartbeat; often benign.

Cause: impulse variations coming into the sinoatrial node from the vagus nerve; electrolyte imbalances.

Contraindications/Indications: consult with client's doctor; any massage should be light and soothing.

Pericarditis — inflammation of the pericardium (sac that surrounds the heart).

Cause: bacterial or viral infection; calcium and fibrous deposits around the heart.

Contraindications/Indications: consult with client's doctor before performing any bodywork; the presence of infection is a contraindication to massage.

Phlebitis — inflammation of a vein; quite common; not very serious in superficial veins; more serious in deep veins.

Cause: unknown (most cases); injury; predisposing factors include obesity and lack of activity.

Contraindications/Indications: do not massage affected area.

Hemorrhoids — a condition characterized by varicose veins of the rectum and anus.

Cause: increased pressure on the veins of the anus; pregnancy.

Contraindications/Indications: do not massage the surrounding gluteal and coccygeal areas.

Coarctation of the aorta — localized narrowing of the aorta; impedes blood flow.

Cause: congenital defect.

Contraindications/Indications: consult with client's doctor.

Aneurysm — a localized bulge in the wall of an artery.

Cause: weakening in the arterial wall.

Contraindications/Indications: avoid the area where the aneurysm is located; avoid abdominal massage.

Murmur — sound heard when blood escapes through a valve of the heart.

Cause: leaky heart valve (congenital condition); previous infection of heart tissue.

Contraindications/Indications: consult with client's doctor; many heart murmurs are benign, but check with client's doctor to be sure.

Myocardial infarction — sudden insufficient blood supply to a segment of heart muscle; results in an area of necrotic cardiac muscle tissue; symptoms include angina, shortness of breath, and radiating pain.

Cause: usually atherosclerosis of the coronary arteries.

Contraindications/Indications: if client has symptoms of infarction, refer to doctor immediately.

Angina pectoris — pain in the chest and arm that may be described as dull, sharp, burning, or aching.

Cause: myocardial ischemia.

Contraindications/Indications: refer to doctor before any bodywork is done; massage should be light and soothing; avoid endangerment areas; avoid abdominal massage, which may increase pressure to the heart.

Heart block — a block in the conduction pathway of the heart; results in uncoordinated contractions of the atria and ventricles.

Cause: damage to a portion of the conduction system in the heart.

Contraindications/Indications: refer to doctor.

Varicose vein — a vein that swells with accumulating blood; condition is usually permanent.

Cause: excessive pressure on the veins causing failure of the one-way valves.

Contraindications/Indications: avoid massage to all affected areas because clots that may form could be broken off into the general circulation.

Arteriosclerosis — hardening of the arteries; decreased blood flow to the brain and extremities may cause dizziness and headaches.

Atherosclerosis — hardening of the arteries resulting from buildup of plaque made of cholesterol and lipids; decrease in elasticity causes narrowing of lumen, leading to decreased blood flow through the artery.

Cause: diabetes; obesity; steroid use; some hereditary metabolic disorders.

Contraindications/Indications: get doctor's approval before proceeding; avoid any deep tissue work; avoid head and neck region.

Raynaud's disease — a condition characterized by peripheral vasoconstriction, most commonly in the digits; most common in women; symptoms include extreme cold, numbness, and pain in the digits; differential diagnoses include scleroderma, thoracic outlet syndrome, stress, and exposure to vibrating machinery.
Cause: unknown.
Contraindications/Indications: massage may increase circulation, reduce associated stress, and relax affected muscles.

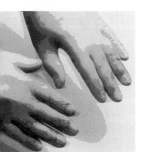

Chapter Thirty-Two

Diseases of the Lymphatic and Immune Systems

Lymphatic System

Elephantiasis — a condition in which blockage of lymphatic vessels results in enormous enlargement of body parts (e.g., legs, scrotum); the end stage of filariasis.
Cause: filarial infection.
Contraindications/Indications: consult client's doctor before performing any bodywork.

Infectious mononucleosis (kissing disease) — a contagious disease spread through direct contact; produces swollen lymph nodes and submandibular glands as well as sore throat, fever, rash, overall fatigue, and an enlarged spleen and liver; very common in young adults and adolescents 15 to 25 years of age.
Cause: Epstein-Barr virus infection.
Contraindications/Indications: all bodywork is contraindicated until the doctor gives approval.

Splenomegaly — enlargement of the spleen; may be up to 10 times the normal size.
Cause: mononucleosis; malaria; toxemia.
Contraindications/Indications: obtain doctor's approval before performing bodywork; avoid the abdominal area, especially around the spleen; all massage should be light.

Hodgkin's disease — a type of malignant lymphoma; causes decreased lymphoid function, which leads to decreased T-cell function and immunodeficiency; progresses in stages; usually arises in cervical lymph nodes; most frequently affects young adults; signs and symptoms include splenomegaly, anemia, fatigue, fever, and overall body wasting.
Cause: cancer in lymphatic structures.
Contraindications/Indications: obtain doctor's approval before performing any bodywork.

Immune System

Rejection — occurs when a transplanted tissue is attacked and broken down by the host's immune system.
Cause: natural immune response involving the production of antibodies, white blood cells, and T cells against foreign tissue.
Contraindications/Indications: consult with client's doctor.

Allergy — hypersensitivity to a particular allergen (foreign agent, food, drug) that is usually harmless; may cause bronchial or sinus congestion, runny nose, pruritus (itching), nausea, or even serious systemic reactions such as anaphylactic shock; affects over 15% of the population of the United States; treatment usually includes antihistamine drugs.

Cause: genetically influenced hypersensitive immune system.

Contraindications/Indications: massage is generally indicated; use caution when the client is on medication or is having an allergic reaction.

Acquired immunodeficiency syndrome (AIDS) — a group of disorders characterized by the destruction of the immune system that leaves the person unable to fight infections and cancer; very high incidence among homosexuals and drug users; mortality rate exceeds 80%; signs and symptoms include fatigue, fever, weight loss, and splenomegaly.

Cause: human immunodeficiency virus (HIV) infection that destroys T helper cells, thus inactivating the immune system; Hodgkin's disease; various other diseases.

Contraindications/Indications: always use universal precautions; obtain doctor's approval and advice.

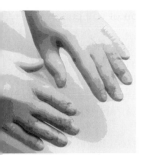

Chapter Thirty-Three

Diseases of the Respiratory System

General Terms

Dyspnea — difficult, labored breathing.
Apnea — absence of breathing.

Disorders

Bronchitis — inflammation (acute or chronic) of the mucous
  membranes in the bronchial tubes of the lung.
  Cause: infection; inhalation of a chemical irritant (e.g.,
    tobacco smoke, dust, car exhaust).
  Contraindications/Indications: can be contagious; refer
    client to a doctor; avoid massage if client has a fever.

> Diseases such as bronchitis
> and emphysema fall under
> the general category of
> **chronic obstructive
> pulmonary disease**
> (COPD).

Emphysema — destruction and enlargement of the alveoli in
  the lung; causes labored breathing and air trapping in
  the lung, leading to "barrel chest" (rounded chest) and
  weight loss.
  Cause: cigarette smoking.
  Contraindications/Indications: massage can relax
    muscles involved in breathing and therefore reduce
    anxiety; consult with client's doctor.

> In some cases of
> **emphysema,** the lung
> capacity is decreased to
> approximately 10% of
> normal. The dramatic
> decrease in the ability to
> maintain normal blood gas
> levels that accompanies
> severe emphysema results in
> early fatigue during simple
> activities such as standing
> and walking across the
> room.

Pneumothorax — accumulation of air in the pleural space
  (i.e., the space between the lung and rib cage); results in
  partial or complete collapse of the lung; commonly
  accompanied by a hemothorax (blood in the pleural space).
  Cause: puncture into the thoracic cavity (e.g., knife wound); fractured or dislocated
    ribs.
  Contraindications/Indications: refer client to a doctor; massage is contraindicated.
Asthma — a disease characterized by episodes ("attacks") of muscle spasm or
  inflammation of the bronchi and bronchiole tubes.
  Cause: allergic response to a particular allergen (e.g., pollen, dust, food, drug);
    emotional or physical stress or strenuous exercise.
  Contraindications/Indications: massage can be very effective in reducing stress; all
    bodywork should be gentle and relaxing.
Tuberculosis — an infectious disease that leads to the development of tubercles (i.e.,
  small masses of bacteria and necrotic tissue surrounded by macrophages) in the
  alveoli of the lung.

Cause: *Mycobacterium tuberculosis* infection acquired by inhalation of the bacteria.
Contraindications/Indications: consult with client's doctor.

Coryza (common cold) — inflammation of the mucous membranes of the upper respiratory tract; signs and symptoms include excessive nasal secretions, tearing, sore throat, hoarse voice, and general malaise; usually lasts about 6 to 7 days.
Cause: viral infection of the upper respiratory tract; most commonly spread by touching the eyes and nose with fingers that have come into contact with an infected surface.
Contraindications/Indications: avoid direct contact with the client (contagious condition); allow symptoms to clear before performing any bodywork.

Pneumonia — inflammation of the bronchioles and alveoli of the lungs.
Cause: bacterial or fungal infection; inhalation of irritating fumes or particles.
Contraindications/Indications: consult with client's doctor; massage during acute stages is contraindicated; massage is beneficial for respiratory muscles and shoulders during the postacute stage; the doctor may advise tapotement to promote expectoration.

Pleurisy (pleuritis) — inflammation of the pleura (i.e, the membrane lining the thoracic cavity); a painful condition made worse by inspiration.
Cause: viral infection; tuberculosis; cancer.
Contraindications/Indications: refer client to a doctor; medical care should precede any bodywork.

Cystic fibrosis — an inherited multisystem disease of the exocrine glands; results in the production of excessive, thick mucus that obstructs the gastrointestinal, respiratory, and urinary systems.
Cause: genetic (1 in 20 Caucasians carry the cystic fibrosis trait).
Contraindications/Indications: avoid the area around the pancreas if inflamed; obtain doctor's approval; tapotement to the chest, light exercise, and bronchodilators increase drainage of the bronchioles.

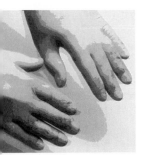

Chapter Thirty-Four

Diseases of the Digestive System

Disorders of the Oral Cavity

Gingivitis — inflammation of the gums.
> **Cause:** accumulation of food between the gums and teeth; bacterial infection; overall poor health; irregular shape, size, and alignment of teeth.
> **Contraindications/Indications:** none.

Periodontitis — inflammation involving the soft tissue (e.g., gums, ligaments) and bone tissue surrounding the teeth; leads to tooth loss.
> **Cause:** residual food; bacterial infection; tartar buildup.
> **Contraindications/Indications:** none.

Canker sores (aphthous ulcers) — small sores that develop in the oral cavity; usually have a yellow or gray center surrounded by a red border; affect approximately 20% of the population of the United States.
> **Cause:** unknown; influenced by emotional stress and poor nutrition.
> **Contraindications/Indications:** avoid pressure around the cheeks and mouth if painful.

Disorders of the Esophagus

Esophagitis — inflammation of the esophagus; usually accompanied by heartburn.
> **Cause:** trauma; infection; irritation from acid reflux or ingestion of hot or spicy food.
> **Contraindications/Indications:** consult with client's doctor before beginning any bodywork; massage of the chest and intercostal muscles can reduce the stress of the condition.

Disorders of the Stomach and Intestines

Gastritis — inflammation of the stomach mucosa.
> **Cause:** exact mechanism is unknown; causative agents include aspirin, alcohol, caffeine, and bacterial toxins.
> **Contraindications/Indications:** avoid the immediate area of the stomach; massage of the thoracic and lumbar spine may relieve tension and anxiety; energy work could also help.

Gastroenteritis — inflammation of the stomach and intestines; leads to abdominal pain, nausea, and diarrhea.

Cause: bacterial or viral infection; allergic reaction; exposure to irritating substances.

Contraindications/Indications: check with the client's doctor before performing bodywork; light, clockwise effleurage to the abdomen to induce relaxation could be beneficial.

Peptic ulcers — ulceration of the mucosa lining the stomach and duodenum (occurs four to five times more frequently in the duodenum); affects about 10% of the total population of the United States.

Cause: *Helicobacter pylori* infection (70% to 80%); use of nonsteroidal anti-inflammatory drugs (e.g., aspirin, ibuprofen, naproxen) [20% to 30%].

Contraindications/Indications: massage of affected area is contraindicated; energy work may be beneficial; massage of reflex areas of the lower spine can help; general massage to reduce stress can also be helpful.

Crohn's disease (regional enteritis) — a disorder involving inflammation of the mucosa, primarily in the ileum of the small intestine, but also in the large intestine; can develop strictures from accumulated scar tissue, which leads to malabsorption of nutrients; signs and symptoms include diarrhea, abdominal pain, nausea, and fever.

Cause: unknown; genetic predisposition suspected.

Contraindications/Indications: obtain doctor's advice before beginning any bodywork; relaxing abdominal massage could be beneficial.

Diverticulosis — a condition characterized by the presence of sac-like bulges (diverticula) or herniations, usually in the muscular wall of the descending colon; if these diverticula become inflamed, the condition is known as diverticulitis.

Cause: weakness of the intestinal wall, usually due to decreased dietary fiber.

Contraindications/Indications: gentle, clockwise massage can relieve the symptoms.

Irritable bowel syndrome — a disorder characterized by recurrent abdominal pain, cramps, and alternating diarrhea and constipation.

Cause: unknown; often associated with emotional stress.

Contraindications/Indications: gentle, clockwise massage can relieve the symptoms; massage of the lumbar, gluteal, and thigh muscles can help alleviate referred pain.

Disorders of the Liver

Hepatitis A — inflammation of the liver tissue; virus is transmitted via the fecal-oral route (e.g., eating or drinking contaminated water or milk, eating seafood from contaminated waters); usually accompanied by headache, nausea, vomiting, jaundice, dark urine, clay-colored stool, and abdominal pain and tenderness; does not cause chronic disease or a carrier state.

Cause: viral infection.

Contraindications/Indications: hepatitis A should be treated medically before performing any bodywork; doctor's approval and advice should be received before performing any bodywork.

Hepatitis B — inflammation of the liver tissue; considered more serious than hepatitis A; transmitted by body fluids or blood products (i.e., whole blood, blood plasma, saliva, urine, semen, tears); signs and symptoms are similar to hepatitis A; can cause chronic disease and a carrier state in about 10% to 15% of cases.

Cause: viral infection.

Contraindications/Indications: hepatitis B should be treated medically before performing any bodywork; doctor's approval and advice should be received before performing any bodywork.

Hepatitis C — inflammation of the liver tissue; produces the same signs and symptoms as hepatitis A and B; transmitted by blood products and contaminated needles; responsible for 50% of chronic hepatitis cases and produces a carrier state.
  Cause: viral infection.
  Contraindications/Indications: hepatitis C should be treated medically before performing bodywork; doctor's approval and advice should be received before performing any bodywork.
Jaundice — a condition in which there is yellow coloration of the skin as a result of the accumulation of bilirubin (a waste product of hemoglobin breakdown) in the blood.
  Cause: excessive red blood cell breakdown; liver failure; an obstruction in the bile ducts.
  Contraindications/Indications: refer client to a doctor before beginning any bodywork.
Cirrhosis of the liver — long-term necrosis of the liver leading to destruction of hepatocytes and accumulation of fibrous scar tissue; some areas of hepatocytes remain and regenerate, developing into nodules (i.e., cells surrounded by fibrous tissue).
  Cause: alcoholism; gallstones leading to bile obstructions; hepatitis A, B, or C.
  Contraindications/Indications: avoid abdominal massage; massage of lower extremities may reduce related edema, but be cautious because excessive fluid movement may stress the liver.

Disorders of the Gallbladder

Cholecystitis — acute or chronic inflammation of the gallbladder; common signs and symptoms include indigestion, vomiting, fever, and tenderness in the right upper quadrant of the abdomen.
  Cause: formation of gallstones (cholelithiasis) that block the flow of bile from the gallbladder.
  Contraindications/Indications: avoid deep massage over the abdomen; general massage of thoracic and lumbar regions relieves tension.

Disorders of the Appendix

Appendicitis — inflammation of the vermiform appendix.
  Cause: obstruction in the small lumen of the appendix leading to increased pressure, ischemia, and eventually bacterial infection.
  Contraindications/Indications: acute appendicitis can be life threatening and needs immediate medical attention; massage is contraindicated even with minor tenderness around the appendix; energy techniques should be used with caution.

Eating Disorders

Anorexia nervosa — an eating disorder characterized by self-starvation, an intense abhorrence for obesity, and often an obsession with exercise; affects 20 times more females than males; has a 5% mortality rate.
  Cause: psychologic self-perception of being overweight.

> **Anorexia nervosa** and **bulimia nervosa** are often accompanied by dehydration; vitamin, mineral, and electrolyte deficiencies; hypoglycemia; anemia; amenorrhea; and urinary and bowel difficulties.

Contraindications/Indications: massage can assist in relieving emotional stress; it would be appropriate to refer client to a doctor.

Bulimia nervosa — an eating disorder characterized by binge eating followed by self-induced vomiting; often called "binge-purge syndrome."

Cause: psychologic self-perception of being overweight.

Contraindications/Indications: massage can assist in relieving emotional stress; it would be appropriate to refer client to a doctor.

Other Disorders

Peritonitis — inflammation of the peritoneum (i.e., the lining of the abdominal cavity).

Cause: ruptured peptic ulcer; ruptured appendix; diverticulitis; peritoneal dialysis; bacterial or viral infection.

Contraindications/Indications: this condition can be life threatening; medical attention must be given before performing any bodywork.

Hernia — protrusion of an organ through an abnormal opening in a tissue of the body.

Cause: lifting; pushing; coughing; straining; congenital defect.

Contraindications/Indications: do not massage affected area; refer client to a doctor.

Hiatal hernia — herniation through the esophageal hiatus (i.e., the opening in the diaphragm that allows the esophagus to pass through), usually by the fundus of the stomach.

Median/epigastric hernia — herniation through the linea alba (i.e., the "white line" of the tendon at the center of the rectus abdominis muscle), usually by the omentum or connective tissue.

Inguinal hernia — herniation through the inguinal ligament (i.e., the ligament connecting the anterior superior iliac spine to the pubic spine), usually by the small intestine.

Umbilical hernia — herniation in the umbilical region, usually due to a congenital deformity.

Femoral hernia — herniation through the femoral ring into the femoral canal (i.e., the canal that contains the femoral artery).

Heartburn — pain or burning sensation in the lower region of the chest.

Cause: regurgitation of gastric juice from the stomach into the esophagus.

Contraindications/Indications: do not massage the upper abdominal area; downward effleurage may soothe the stomach and abdominal muscles and reduce the regurgitation of gastric juice.

Diarrhea — frequent passage of watery stools; sometimes accompanied by nausea, vomiting, cramps, and malaise; leads to dehydration if left untreated, so plenty of fluids are essential.

Cause: viral or bacterial infection; food poisoning; metabolic disorders; irritable bowel syndrome; colitis.

Contraindications/Indications: massage is indicated.

Constipation — difficulty in having bowel movements.

Cause: very hard stools; decreased dietary fiber; dehydration.

Contraindications/Indications: massage of the abdomen in a clockwise pattern can facilitate peristalsis.

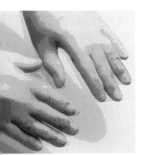

Chapter Thirty-Five

Diseases of the Urinary System

General Terms

Dialysis — artificial filtering of the blood using a semipermeable membrane and dialysis fluid (i.e., fluid that is isotonic to normal blood); used to filter out waste products from the blood of an individual with renal failure.

    Contraindications/Indications: consult with a doctor before performing bodywork.

    Hemodialysis — dialysis performed by a machine that removes arterial blood and cycles it through one side of a chamber that is separated by a semipermeable membrane from the other side, which is filled with dialysis fluid; waste products diffuse from the blood into the dialysis fluid, and any substances in which the blood is deficient diffuse from the dialysis fluid into the blood.

    Peritoneal dialysis — a process that operates on the same principle as hemodialysis but uses the peritoneum (i.e., the membrane lining the abdominal cavity) as the semipermeable membrane; dialysis fluid is infused into the abdominal cavity through a catheter and allowed to remain there approximately 30 to 45 minutes before being drained away; waste products diffuse from the mesenteric blood vessels, through the peritoneum, and into the dialysis fluid.

> Although both **hemodialysis** and **peritoneal dialysis** are effective means of filtering blood for chronic or acute renal failure, each has advantages and disadvantages. Hemodialysis is quicker and safer, but it is expensive and requires the assistance of a trained technician to operate the machine. Peritoneal dialysis is cheaper, requires less equipment, and can be performed without assistance; however, it takes about six times longer and carries a high risk of subsequent infection (peritonitis).

Disorders

Nephritis — acute or chronic inflammation of the kidney.

    Cause: bacterial or viral infection triggering an immune response.

    Contraindications/Indications: it is best to get the doctor's advice before performing bodywork; increased circulation may aggravate the condition.

Urethritis — inflammation of the urethra; usually impedes the outflow of urine.

    Cause: bacterial or viral infection (sexually transmitted diseases).

    Contraindications/Indications: massage is indicated; avoid the lower abdomen.

Cystitis — inflammation of the urinary bladder and ureters; characterized by frequent, painful urination and blood in the urine; more common in females.

    Cause: microbial infection.

Contraindications/Indications: massage is indicated; avoid the lower abdomen.

Urolithiasis — a condition in which kidney stones (calculi) develop in the renal calyces or pelvis.

Cause: increased calcium in the blood.

Contraindications/Indications: obtain the doctor's advice; massage is generally indicated; use caution around the kidneys and lower abdomen.

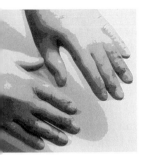

Chapter Thirty-Six

Diseases of the Reproductive System

General Terms

Vasectomy (deferentectomy) — surgery in which the vas deferens (ductus deferens) is severed and tied off, rendering the male sterile.

Impotence — inability of a male to maintain an erection or achieve ejaculation.

Cryptorchism — failure of one testis or both testes to descend into the scrotum during fetal development.

Phimosis — tightness of the foreskin (prepuce) around the glans penis.

Hysterectomy — surgical removal of the uterus.

Radical mastectomy — complete surgical removal of the breast and surrounding tissue, including the pectoralis major muscle.

> Edema of the upper extremity frequently accompanies a mastectomy and is caused by damage to the blood and lymph vessels. Massage helps tremendously to remove excess fluids from the tissue.

Disorders

Uterine fibroid — a benign tumor of the smooth muscle in the uterus; occurs in 20% to 30% of women older than 30 years of age; may enlarge during pregnancy and shrink after menopause; most are asymptomatic, but may contribute to infertility and spontaneous abortion.

Ectopic pregnancy [*ektopios = out of place*] — implantation of the fertilized ovum (egg) outside of the uterus (e.g., in the uterine tubes or on the peritoneum).

Placenta previa — a condition in which the placenta is attached to the uterine lining in the lower portion of the uterus; can cause abruptio placentae and necessitate a cesarean section to spare the mother's or baby's life.

Abruptio placentae — a condition in which the placenta prematurely separates from the wall of the uterus; leads to bleeding and fetal distress.

Infertility — inability of fertilization to take place.
    Cause: in the male, inadequate sperm production, alcoholism, dietary insufficiencies, excessive body heat, x-ray exposure; in the female, hormonal imbalances, obstructions in the uterine tubes, abnormal ovulation.
    Contraindications/Indications: refer client to a doctor.

Sterility — permanent state of being unable to reproduce.
    Cause: degeneration of the gonads or other sexual organs; genetic predisposition.
    Contraindications/Indications: refer client to a doctor.

Orchitis — inflammation of the testis.
    Cause: most commonly from mumps, a transient viral infection.
    Contraindications/Indications: refer client to a doctor.

Genital herpes — a common sexually transmitted disease; mostly seen in young adults; infects nearly all of the external genitalia in both males and females; characterized by vesicles that ulcerate and produce shallow lesions; can be transmitted to newborns as they pass through the birth canal; systemic forms of herpes can be fatal, particularly in newborns and premature infants.
   Cause: herpes simplex type 2 virus infection.
   Contraindications/Indications: refer client to a doctor.
Prostatitis — inflammation of the prostate gland; can be acute or chronic.
   Cause: in most cases the cause is uncertain; can be a bacterial infection.
   Contraindications/Indications: refer client to a doctor.
   Acute prostatitis — common in young, sexually active males; accompanied by a swollen, tender prostate gland, fever, and painful urination.
   Chronic prostatitis — a common condition of middle-aged and elderly males; a swollen prostate gland and painful urination are common symptoms; can be accompanied by lower back pain, urine retention, or even kidney infections.
Vaginitis — inflammation of the vagina.
   Cause: bacterial, fungal, or viral infection; trauma.
   Contraindications/Indications: refer client to a doctor.
Salpingitis — inflammation of the uterine (fallopian) tubes.
   Cause: bacterial or viral infection; trauma.
   Contraindications/Indications: refer client to a doctor.
Mastitis — inflammation of the breast; accompanied by swelling of the breast tissue, pain, and swelling of lymph nodes in the armpit region; common during the first 2 months of lactation.
   Cause: bacterial infection; trauma.
   Contraindications/Indications: refer client to a doctor.
Amenorrhea — absence or abnormal cessation of menstruation.
   Cause: menopause; pregnancy; lactation; anorexia nervosa; athletic training.
   Contraindications/Indications: refer client to a doctor.
Dysmenorrhea — painful or difficult menstruation; usually accompanied by severe menstrual cramps.
   Cause: hormonal imbalances; endometriosis; uterine tumor.
   Contraindications/Indications: massage may be beneficial to reduce circulatory congestion and associated pain; energy work may be effective.
Endometriosis — a condition in which endometrial tissue is found outside of the interior lining of the uterus (e.g., in the ovaries, outer layer of the uterus, abdominal wall, urinary bladder); affects about 15% of women; signs and symptoms include dysmenorrhea, painful urination, and infertility.
   Cause: fragments of endometrial tissue forced backward through the uterine tubes during menstruation.
   Contraindications/Indications: refer client to a doctor.
Pelvic inflammatory disease (PID) — inflammation of the female reproductive organs in the pelvis; symptoms include low back pain, fever, and vaginal discharge.
   Cause: bacterial infection beginning in the vagina and uterus.
   Contraindications/Indications: refer client to a doctor.
Toxic shock syndrome — shock brought on by acute bacterial infection; usually affects menstruating women who use high-absorbency tampons; onset is sudden and accompanied by fever, aching joints and muscles, sore throat, and diarrhea; can be fatal.
   Cause: toxins produced by *Staphylococcus aureus,* a widespread bacteria that is normal flora in many tissues of healthy individuals.
   Contraindications/Indications: refer client to a doctor.

Breast cancer (carcinoma of the breast) — the most common malignant disorder affecting women (10% of women); metastasis occurs through lymph fluid or blood into the lymph nodes, lungs, liver, other glands, and bones; most significant sign is detection of a lump in the breast.

    Cause: linked to a genetic mutation in chromosome 17, but influenced greatly by several environmental factors (e.g., obesity, high levels of estrogens); silicone breast implants are an unlikely cause.

    Contraindications/Indications: refer client to a doctor, particularly if you observe changes in the axillary region.

Uterine cancer (carcinoma of the uterus) — most commonly found in the cervix of the uterus; second most common site of cancer after breast cancer; can be detected early through a Pap smear (i.e., biopsy of cervical tissue).

    Cause: sexual transmission of virus (human papilloma virus); also influenced by environmental factors (e.g., smoking).

    Contraindications/Indications: refer client to a doctor.

Prostate cancer (prostatic carcinoma) — second leading cause of death in the United States after lung cancer; usually affects males older than 70 years of age; accounts for over 20,000 deaths annually in the United States.

    Cause: appears to have a genetic component (incidence is higher in African Americans than in Caucasians); influenced by testosterone.

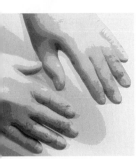

Practice Questions

Clinical Pathology

Multiple Choice Questions

Select the one lettered answer or completion that is best in each case.

1. Which of the following terms is used to describe a condition that is intense, has a sudden onset, and is of short duration?
   A. Endemic
   B. Chronic
   C. Acute
   D. Morbid

2. A pandemic disease affects:
   A. a community
   B. an entire region
   C. the entire world
   D. a continent

3. If the adrenal cortex is producing too much cortisol because of hypersecretion of adrenocorticotropic hormone, which of the following conditions will develop?
   A. Cushing's disease
   B. A goiter
   C. Addison's disease
   D. Dwarfism

4. A spasm in the sternocleidomastoid muscle that causes the head to tilt or rotate to one side is characteristic of:
   A. muscle soreness
   B. torticollis
   C. deficiency of vitamins or minerals in the muscle
   D. muscular dystrophy

5. Virulence refers to:
   A. the ability to kill every living organism present
   B. the ability of an organism to cause a disease
   C. the pattern of development of a certain disease
   D. none of the above

6. Inflammation of the urinary bladder is called:
   A. nephritis
   B. cystitis
   C. pyelonephritis
   D. glomerulonephritis

7. A person who is allergic to bee stings is stung by a bee and experiences a massive release of histamine causing widespread vasodilation and hypotension. This reaction is called:
   A. asthma
   B. septic shock
   C. anaphylactic shock
   D. phlebitis

8. Myalgia means:
   A. nerve pain
   B. muscle pain
   C. muscle spasm
   D. softening of cartilage

9. What kind of immunity is developed when a baby inherits antibodies across the placenta and through the mother's breast milk?
   A. Natural passive immunity
   B. Natural active immunity
   C. Artificial active immunity
   D. Artificial passive immunity

10. Which of the following is a malignant tumor of epithelial tissue?
    A. Carcinoma
    B. Lipoma
    C. Sarcoma
    D. Adenoma

11. The client's emotional state and level of stress both play an important role in the client's overall health.
    A. True
    B. False

12. Which of the following is a metabolic disorder involving the development of tophi (i.e., masses of uric acid crystals surrounded by macrophages) in and around joints?
    A. Osgood-Schlatter disease
    B. Bursitis
    C. Rheumatoid arthritis
    D. Gout

13. Failure of one testis or both testes to descend into the scrotum during fetal development is called:
    A. phimosis
    B. cryptorchism
    C. orchitis
    D. mastitis

14. Which of the following diseases is characterized by deposition of collagen in the skin, lungs, heart, kidneys, and gastrointestinal tract?
    A. Urticaria
    B. Pruritus
    C. Decubitus ulcers
    D. Scleroderma

15. Which of the following terms is used to refer to an abnormality that is outward and observable?
A. Diagnosis
B. Sign
C. Symptom
D. Syndrome

16. Which of the following conditions is characterized by the development of excessive pressure in the eye?
A. Cataract
B. Strabismus
C. Hyperopia
D. Glaucoma

17. What is the function of histamine?
A. Vasodilation
B. Production of antibodies
C. Increased blood vessel permeability
D. Both A and C
E. Both A and B

18. Increased calcium in the blood leads to the development of kidney stones. This condition is called:
A. glomerulonephritis
B. pyelonephritis
C. urolithiasis
D. prostatitis

19. Which of the following is a viral infection characterized by the development of pustules along a dermatomal pattern?
A. Shingles
B. Impetigo
C. Chickenpox
D. Carcinoma

20. Thrombocytopenia is:
A. an abnormal increase in the number of red blood cells
B. an abnormal decrease in the number of circulating platelets
C. a disease characterized by an increase in immature, ineffective white blood cells
D. the condition resulting from inadequate delivery of oxygenated blood to the tissues

21. Hardening of the arteries due to a buildup of plaque made of cholesterol and lipids is called:
A. heart block
B. atherosclerosis
C. heart murmur
D. varicosity

22. A myoma is a tumor of:
A. nerve tissue
B. cartilaginous tissue
C. muscle tissue
D. eye tissue

23. Necrosis refers to:
   A. a lack of blood supply
   B. a free-floating blood clot
   C. cell or tissue death
   D. a decrease in the number of circulating white blood cells

24. The absence or cessation of menstruation is called:
   A. sterility
   B. vaginitis
   C. dysmenorrhea
   D. amenorrhea

25. Tinea cruris is also called:
   A. shingles
   B. athlete's foot
   C. jock itch
   D. hives

26. Which of the following disorders is caused by decreased production of dopamine in the midbrain and is characterized by impairment of motor functions, tremors, body rigidity, poor balance, tiredness, weakness, slow speech, and a shuffling gait?
   A. Parkinson's disease
   B. Alzheimer's disease
   C. Cerebral palsy
   D. Bell's palsy

27. Which of the following is a predisposing factor of disease?
   A. Lifestyle
   B. Nutrition/diet
   C. Age
   D. Preexisting illness
   E. All of the above

28. Which of the following occurs when a transplanted tissue is attacked and broken down by a host's immune system?
   A. Rejection syndrome
   B. An allergy
   C. Acquired immunodeficiency syndrome (AIDS)
   D. Passive, naturally acquired immunity

29. Emphysema is the term used to describe:
   A. a collapsed lung
   B. destruction of the alveoli in the lung
   C. muscle spasms in the bronchiole tubes
   D. none of the above

30. Which of the following is an autoimmune disorder that affects the skin?
   A. Impetigo
   B. Scleroderma
   C. Scabies
   D. Tinea cruris

31. The yellow coloration of the skin that results from the accumulation of bilirubin in the blood is called:
A. pustules
B. cyanosis
C. vesicles
D. jaundice

32. Which of the following diseases is characterized by a deficiency of antidiuretic hormone from the anterior pituitary gland?
A. Cushing's disease
B. Diabetes mellitus
C. Addison's disease
D. Diabetes insipidus

33. Inflammation of the middle ear is properly called:
A. otitis interna
B. otitis media
C. otosclerosis
D. conjunctivitis

34. Which of the following will most likely develop if a person lies in bed without shifting or moving and experiences prolonged pressure over bony prominences?
A. Urticaria
B. Decubitus ulcers
C. Scoliosis
D. Osteomyelitis

35. The eating disorder characterized by self-starvation, an intense abhorrence for obesity, and often an obsession with exercise is called:
A. anorexia nervosa
B. bulimia nervosa
C. urticaria
D. Huntington's disease

36. An osteoma is a tumor of:
A. bone tissue
B. cartilaginous tissue
C. lung tissue
D. skin tissue

37. Which of the following terms refers to inflamed gums?
A. Gingivitis
B. Glossitis
C. Polyps
D. Gastritis

38. Which of the following is a cause of scoliosis?
A. Leg length discrepancy
B. Spina bifida
C. Spinal nerve root damage
D. All of the above

39. A progressive nervous disease characterized by rapid, writhing contortions or rigidity of the muscles in the hands, arms, trunk, and face that leads to total incapacitation and death after about 15 years is:
A. meningitis
B. encephalitis
C. Huntington's disease
D. spina bifida

40. Surgical removal of the uterus is a:
A. hysterectomy
B. vasectomy
C. radical mastectomy
D. deferentectomy

41. Which of the following fractures occurs when a piece of bone is chipped or broken off?
A. Compound
B. Impacted
C. Comminuted
D. Avulsion

42. Which of the following conditions is characterized by pain in the chest that radiates down the left arm?
A. Angina pectoris
B. Arrhythmia
C. Heart murmur
D. Phlebitis

43. Which of the following types of burns is characterized by open wounds with black charring and white patches of necrotic tissue?
A. Third-degree burn
B. Second-degree burn
C. First-degree burn
D. Fourth-degree burn

44. A history of abnormal wear and tear on the joints and deterioration of the articular cartilage suggests a diagnosis of:
A. Osgood-Schlatter disease
B. osteoporosis
C. osteoarthritis
D. gout

45. Hodgkin's disease is:
A. an infection of filarial worms in the lymphatic system that causes lymph blockage and enlargement of body parts
B. a contagious disease spread by direct contact that produces swollen lymph nodes and submandibular glands
C. a type of malignant lymphoma that causes decreased lymphoid function and immunodeficiency
D. enlargement of the spleen

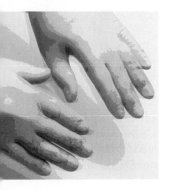

Part III
Massage Therapy and Bodywork: Theory, Assessment, and Application

Chapter Thirty-Seven

Introduction to Bodywork

Definitions

Massage

According to the **Utah Massage Practice Act of 1995,** massage is the practice whereby a person, either by the use of the hands or a mechanical or electrical apparatus, administers to another person **effleurage** (stroking), **friction** (rubbing), **pétrissage** (kneading), **tapotement** (percussion) and **vibration** (shaking or trembling), or variations of these techniques. It also includes the use of rehabilitative procedures involving the muscles by nonintrusive means and without spinal manipulation. The practice of massage may also include the use of oil rubs; heat lamps; salt glows; hot and cold packs; or tub, shower, steam, or cabinet baths. Massology is the study of massage and its techniques. Note that each state or political subdivision has a different definition for massage, so contact the local authorities that regulate this profession in your area.

The English word "massage" has ancient and international origins:

Masso or **massein** (Greek) means "to touch or handle, to knead or squeeze."
Massa (Latin) also means "to touch or handle, to knead or squeeze."
Mass or **mass'h** (Arabic) means "to press softly."
Champo or **tshanpau** (Hindi) means "to massage" or "to press."
Masser (French, from the Arabic or Latin) means "to massage."

Massage Technician or Therapist

According to the **Utah Massage Practice Act of 1995,** a massage technician (or therapist) is a person who engages in or teaches the practice of massage for a fee, gratuity, or free demonstration. Other acceptable terms include **massologist, masseuse** (female), **masseur** (male), and **myomassologist.** Note that each state or political subdivision has a different definition, so contact the local authorities that regulate this profession in your area.

History of Massage

Background

Since the dawn of time it has been a basic, instinctive reaction to place a hand over or to rub a part of the body that is injured. Every culture has had some type of medicine man, shaman, or tribal "witch doctor" who assisted the healing process with massage, herbs, oils, and forms of energy work. Typically, these healing practices were accompanied with pomp and ceremony to promote the mystical and powerful "aura" of the healer. Healers were also given great power and authority, and were considered religious figures because of the powers they claimed from the gods. Even in some current cultures, those that have "healing powers" are revered and set apart.

China

The oldest and most well known of all forms of ancient medicine comes from the Chinese. *The Cong Fau of Tao-Tse,* written in approximately 3000 B.C. and one of the earliest documents ever discovered, describes the foundation for Chinese **amma** (or **anma**) and provides us with the earliest references to the concepts of acupuncture, energy meridians, and acupressure massage.

The early Chinese considered the body a temple not to be defiled. Therefore, doctors were forced to diagnose and treat the body from the only acceptable access areas: the hands, feet, and head. To accomplish this they had to develop, through trial and error, the use of all five senses plus a sixth sense needed to diagnose and treat each problem they encountered. Through this process, the concepts relating to energy meridians were born.

Over the centuries, Chinese medicine evolved into the modern-day concept of keeping the body healthy by promoting balance in the individual's physical, emotional, and spiritual environment. Modern Chinese medicine still uses treatments and medicines that are hundreds of years old, but also provides Western allopathic medical care in the top hospitals. Doctors who specialize in massage (Tui Na) techniques are also an integral part of Chinese medicine.

India

The concepts of Ayurvedic medicine were developed in ancient India. The *Ayur-Veda* ("The Art of Life") is a sacred book of the Hindus that dates to about 1800 B.C. Although thousands of miles from China, the Hindus also found that health is dictated by an individual's physical, emotional, and spiritual environment. According to Ayurvedic philosophies, everything is energetic in nature and interacts energetically with everything else. Therefore, health is influenced by a person's total environment. This belief encompasses all aspects of life (e.g., clothing colors, furniture arrangement) as necessary to promote the most beneficial prana (energy) required for good health.

The concepts of chakra, kundalini, and other energies are the basis for this type of medicine. With the help of pioneers such as Dr. Deepak Chopra and his teaching of these ideas and their relationship to science, American society is just now becoming aware of these concepts.

Japan

The Japanese adopted many practices from Chinese amma around the sixth century A.D. In Chinese acupuncture, over 2000 points are documented for use in treatment. The Japanese simplified this healing practice into a modality that uses only the most effective 660 points (tsubos) in what we now know as **Shiatsu** (see Chapter 45 for a description of Shiatsu).

Greece and Rome

Based on many of the writings found dating around 300 B.C., massage was a primary ingredient in the practice of medicine in Greek and Roman cultures. War was important in these cultures to demonstrate Greek and Roman superiority. To keep military forces strong, massage was used to rehabilitate injured and fatigued soldiers so they could return to battle as soon as possible. Even in the sporting arenas, gladiators were treated with massage for the same reason.

Some of the most famous Greek physicians, historians, and philosophers, such as Asclepiades, Herodotus, and Homer, were known for their writings about massage and nutrition. Famous Roman authors who discussed massage in their writings include Celsus, Galen, Plato, and Cicero. Hippocrates (460 to 380 B.C.), considered the "Father of Medicine," emphasized in his writings the value of massage in medical treatment.

It is recorded that Julius Caesar demanded a daily massage to maintain his youth and vitality. Because the Romans considered themselves the supreme race, all citizens were allowed the privilege of receiving massage and therapeutic baths, regardless of their station in life.

Dark Ages

During the Dark Ages (around 476 to 1450 A.D.), religion assumed a primary role in everyday life, with religious organizations and their officials taking on great power. Fear of the sciences and of learning, including healing arts and practices, was instilled in the people, who were taught to focus instead on saving their souls through religious leaders. All those associated with the sciences and healing were persecuted and forced to go underground. As a result, much information was destroyed or lost, including many writings on massage and other healing practices.

Renaissance

After about 1450 A.D., the arts and sciences were revived when religious authority was overshadowed by the changes brought about by inventions such as the printing press. During this time, education and research became much more accessible and people began to discuss their work and communicate across wider distances, giving rise to modern science and eventually leading to the information age. Spiritual matters were left to the religious community, while scientists began to catalog and take control of physical matters.

Recent Years

During World Wars I and II and other early 20th century military actions taken by the United States, massage was used to rehabilitate weary soldiers. Nurses were required to receive 70 hours of massage training. Eventually, massage became more mainstream, and at the 1984 Olympic Games in Los Angeles, massage was officially offered for the first time to the Olympic athletes of the United States.

Major Contributors in the History of Massage

Ambroise Paré (1517 to 1590)

Ambroise Paré is noted as the founder of modern surgery for his work on the ligation of arteries. He was a French barber and surgeon who touted the healing benefits of massage in his writings.

Per Henrik Ling (1776 to 1839)

Per Henrik Ling was a physiologist and fencing master who developed the movements known as Swedish remedial gymnastics, or Swedish massage. In 1813 the Swedish government created the Royal Swedish Central Institute of Gymnastics as a result of the successful work that was being done in the medical arena.

Dr. Johann Mezger (1839 to 1909)

Dr. Mezger is credited with developing the fundamentals of rehabilitation, in what is now known as **physical therapy.** He also codified the familiar French terminology of Swedish massage (e.g., effleurage, pétrissage).

Dr. S. Weir Mitchell

Dr. Mitchell, a Pennsylvania physician, introduced massage in the United States in 1870.

Dr. Douglas O. Graham

Dr. Graham of Boston published one of the first papers in English on massage in 1874. He continued actively writing on the subject until 1925, and was one of the founding members of the American Physical Education Society. His *Treatise on Massage, Its History, Mode of Application and Effects* (1884) got the attention of the American medical profession and created an awareness of the potential of massage in healing.

Albert J. Hoffa

Albert J. Hoffa, a German physician, wrote *Technik der Massage* (1900), in which he described a technique of massaging the body in anatomical segments. He believed in short massage sessions.

Dr. John Harvey Kellogg

Dr. Kellogg prescribed massage as part of the treatment for patients at his Battle Creek Sanitarium in Michigan during the early 20th century.

Mary McMillan

Mary McMillan, Chief Aide at Walter Reed Army Hospital in 1918, became Director of Physiotherapy at Harvard Medical School. She wrote extensively on the value of massage and therapeutic exercise in physiotherapy, describing five basic massage strokes, each having a specific application and with the focus of promoting lymph flow toward the heart. Mary McMillan was one of the founders of the American Physical Therapy Association and served as its first president in 1921.

Elizabeth Dicke

In the 1940s, Elizabeth Dicke developed a connective tissue massage technique called bindegewebsmassage, in which she postulates that certain surface areas of the body, via the dermatomes, have a direct relationship to certain viscera and to the autonomic and central nervous systems. She created a treatment program, widely used in Germany and other areas of Europe, to directly affect certain conditions.

Harold D. Storms

Harold D. Storms published an article in 1944 describing the benefits and effects of **friction,** a massage stroke in which tissue is manipulated parallel to the muscle fibers.

James Cyriax

James Cyriax described his concept of **deep transverse friction techniques** in his *Textbook of Orthopaedic Medicine,* volume 11 (1977). The techniques focus on slow, unidirectional stroking, working the proximal limb before the distal. The basic effects are to broaden tissues, break down adhesions, and restore mobility. These friction techniques are well known in sports massage (see Chapter 45 for a further discussion of sports massage).

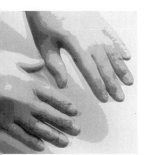

Chapter Thirty-Eight

Assessment

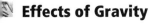

Effects of Gravity

Gravity and Posture

Gravity is a constant force that usually works against proper body posture. Many postural disorders (e.g., kyphosis, "forward head") occur because something has decreased the body's ability to overcome the force of gravity. Because of the large number of postural disorders and the detailed information needed to understand postural deformity due to gravity, all further information is contained in Chapter 25.

Gravity in Massage

Gravity can be used to the advantage of the bodyworker in many ways. For example, when giving a massage, **positioning** of the client is important to **minimize the amount of unnecessary muscle activity;** this is one reason why lying prone or supine is often beneficial.

Circulatory considerations

Gravity has an important effect on **blood and fluid movement** in the body.

Standing
When a person stands up, gravity draws blood from the upper portions of the body down to the lower extremities. If the body does not adapt quickly enough to adjust blood flow, the person will become light-headed and faint.

Stroking
When using massage strokes to reduce inflammation, the inflamed part of the body can be elevated above the heart so that gravity will help draw fluid out of the extremity.

Palpation

Palpation requires the ability to differentiate, compare, and assess many different qualities of the body through touch. Our bodies are innately able to "feel" many different conditions using countless sensory receptors (e.g., nerve receptors, sensory or afferent nerves) that transmit information to the brain for recognition and assessment. Experience is the greatest teacher in the skill of palpation, which is a valuable tool that can dramatically enhance the effects and success of treatment.

Bodywork practitioners develop palpation skills to distinguish basic conditions, such as:

1. Tension
2. Temperature
3. Texture
4. Movements
5. Pulses
6. Adhesions
7. Energy flows and blocks
8. Pain levels

The most common focus areas to understand treatment needs for specific conditions are:

Anatomical systems (i.e., skin, fascia, tendons, ligaments, muscles, blood vessels, lymph nodes, and bones)
Body rhythms (i.e., heartbeat, respiration, cranial rhythms)
Energies in and around the body

Somatic Holding Patterns (see Chapter 40)

Visual Cues in Assessment

Assessment Versus Diagnosis

Because diagnosis (i.e., the identification of a disease based on its signs and symptoms) and treatment are deemed medical terms when related to medical conditions, they are considered outside of the scope of practice for massage therapists. It is important to note that an assessment (i.e., an evaluation in which one examines or judges a situation) should not be misinterpreted as a diagnosis. The difference is that massage therapists "assess" the client's condition for their own purpose in determining a course of action.

Reason For Assessment

1. Design the most appropriate massage session
2. Refer the client to another health care or medical professional

Visual Cues

The most effective assessment includes watching the client walk in the door, interviewing the client, and then continuing a visual scan of the client's body during treatment. Items that a skilled bodyworker can use to visually assess a client include:

> It is wise to always write specific observations in the client's SOAP (subjective, objective, assessment, plan) notes.

1. **Gait or walking pattern**—Is each movement smooth, balanced, and symmetrical?
2. **Posture**—What kind of posture does the client assume (see Chapter 40)?
3. **Basic body structure**—What kind of basic body structure does the client have? Does the client have any obvious deformities (e.g., uneven shoulders or hips, lordosis, kyphosis, scoliosis, visceroptosis, "washboard spine")?
4. **Movement patterns or restrictions**—Does the client exhibit any range of motion deficits or restrictions that may involve a joint or any of the surrounding muscles, tendons, or ligaments?
5. **Eyes**—Does the client keep good eye contact?

6. **Visible pathologic conditions**—Does the client have any visible condition (e.g., varicose veins, bruises, inflammation)?
7. **Breathing**—Is the client's respiration (e.g., rhythm, depth) normal?
8. **Sympathetic or parasympathetic condition**—Sympathetic: Is the client anxious, angry, excited, agitated, or restless? Parasympathetic: Is the client relaxed, calm, content, or depressed?
9. **Emotional condition (or state of mind)**—Can you deduce any more about how the client may be feeling from how the client looks?
10. **Physical condition**—How much "energy" does the client portray? Does the client appear to be energetic or tired?

Western Medical Approaches

It is valuable to understand basic medical assessment techniques in order to add any information gathered for the client's medical history. This adds in creating a better assessment and treatment plan.

Diagnosis

X-ray — an imaging procedure that uses electromagnetic radiation; used to penetrate tissues and identify dense tissue (e.g., bone).

Computed tomography (CT) scan — an imaging procedure that uses electromagnetic radiation similar to that used in X-rays; used to examine the soft tissue of a specific region (e.g., brain).

Magnetic resonance imaging (MRI) — an imaging procedure that uses an electromagnetic field; provides the most accurate and detailed view of all tissue layers in the body.

Biopsy — collection of a small amount of tissue or fluid from the body to examine under a microscope; used to determine the presence of a disease (e.g., cancer).

Complete blood count (CBC) — a common laboratory procedure that involves counting the red blood cells, white blood cells, and platelets from a sample of an individual's blood; used mostly to determine diseases or problems involving red blood cells (e.g., anemia) or white blood cells (e.g., infection, mononucleosis, leukemia).

Urinalysis — a common laboratory procedure to examine the appearance and content of a sample of urine; used to screen for abnormal contents such as blood cells, bacteria, glucose, and other indicators of disease or organ malfunction.

Treatment

Antibiotics — drugs (e.g., penicillin) that destroy, break down, or limit the growth of a living bacterium; used to fight infection in the body.

Surgery — the branch of medicine that deals with treatment of injury and disease using physical operation; used to repair damaged organs or remove diseased tissue or a malignant growth.

Chemotherapy — a form of treatment that involves the use of chemical agents; most commonly used to treat cancer.

Radiotherapy (or radiation therapy) — a form of treatment that involves the use of radiation from radioactive materials; most commonly used to treat cancer.

Nonsteroidal anti-inflammatory drugs (NSAIDs) — a classification of common drugs (e.g., aspirin, ibuprofen, naproxen) that are used to reduce inflammation and pain.

Structural Compensatory Patterns

Because there are so many different ways that the body can compensate, only a brief review of some of the main compensations is presented here.

Alignment — the natural position of a bone or limb as it relates to gravity; joints that are required to function out of their normal position will often become misaligned.

Hypermobility — a condition in which a joint has more range of motion than would normally be permitted; usually associated with lax ligaments.

Hypomobility — a condition in which a joint has less range of motion than would normally be permitted; usually associated with tight ligaments or **contractures** (i.e., shortening of soft tissue structures around a joint).

Substitution — an attempt of one muscle to function in place of another muscle that fails to perform because of pain or weakness; often results in faulty movement patterns; can lead to unbalanced or strained muscles.

Interview Techniques

Review Intake Forms

The intake form is the most important tool to help you determine the proper treatment for an individual. It serves as an evaluation of the client's past medical history along with the client's current condition and needs. If you feel it is necessary and appropriate, it is equally important to ask further questions of the client about medical history and personal needs before beginning treatment.

Listen

The most important interview technique is listening. Communication can come in subtle ways, so pay attention to details, such as voice intonation and pauses.

> Sometimes reading between the lines is a valuable skill to have when forming an evaluation of current needs or determining probable cause and contributing factors. This applies to client intake forms as well as interviewing.

Observe

Observe the client's body language. Does the client's body posture express more of the client's true condition or state? The client may be communicating more than is readily apparent.

Ask Questions

Ask questions that promote subjective and objective answers. For example, "How do you feel?" and "What was your experience?" are good questions to ask because they create opportunities for a more in-depth look at the condition.

Prepare For Treatment

A good interview will lead you to suspect a reason or cause for the accompanying symptoms. Begin your treatment with the intent to explore with your hands the most likely reason for the conditions you discovered in your interview. This allows the practitioner to use physical assessment to validate or augment the interview assessment, thus enhancing the treatment. Remember to keep an open mind.

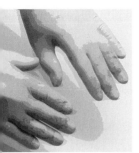

Chapter Thirty-Nine

Application: Precautions

Sites to Avoid (Endangerment Sites)

Certain areas of the body require special precautions because of underlying anatomical structures that could be prone to injury under certain circumstances. In most of these areas, major nerves, vessels, arteries, or organs are relatively close to the surface. Massage may be contraindicated in these areas due to possible injury. Some areas may be contraindicated for Swedish or deep tissue work whereas energy techniques may be beneficial. Following are the areas of concern and the structures involved.

Anterior triangle of the neck — the region bordered by the sternocleidomastoid muscle, mandible, and trachea.

    Contains: carotid artery, jugular vein, vagus nerve, submandibular gland, and cervical lymph nodes.

Posterior triangle of the neck — the region bordered by the sternocleidomastoid muscle, trapezius muscle, and clavicle.

    Contains: nerve roots that form the brachial plexus, subclavian artery, brachiocephalic and jugular veins, and cervical lymph nodes.

Inferior to the ear — the notch posterior and inferior to the ear.

    Contains: external carotid artery, styloid process of the temporal bone, and facial nerve.

Axilla — armpit.

    Contains: axillary, median, radial, musculocutaneous, and ulnar nerves; axillary artery; basilic vein; and axillary lymph nodes.

Medial brachium — upper, inner arm between the biceps and triceps (medial head) muscles.

    Contains: ulnar, median, and musculocutaneous nerves; brachial artery; basilic vein; and lymph nodes.

Cubital area of the elbow — anterior aspect of the elbow.

    Contains: median nerve, radial and ulnar arteries, and median cubital vein.

Ulnar notch of the elbow — posterior elbow; also called the "funny bone."

    Contains: ulnar nerve.

Abdomen — upper abdomen, under the ribs.

    Contains: liver and gallbladder on the right side, spleen on the left side, and the aorta in the center (deep).

Back (upper lumbar region) — region inferior to the ribs and lateral to the spine.

    Contains: kidneys.

> Do not perform percussion over the kidneys.

Sciatic notch — the indentation in the pelvic bones located deep to the gluteus maximus muscle.

   Contains: sciatic nerve.

Femoral triangle — the region bordered by the sartorius muscle, adductor longus muscle, and inguinal ligament.

   Contains: femoral nerve, femoral artery and vein, great saphenous vein, and inguinal lymph nodes.

Popliteal fossa — the space posterior to the knee and bordered by the heads of the gastrocnemius muscle and distal hamstring muscles.

   Contains: popliteal artery and vein, tibial nerve, and common peroneal nerve.

Universal Precautions

The following procedures are used when conditions require contact with any body fluid (i.e., blood, urine, sweat, tears, saliva, and semen). The precautions include proper gloving, masking, and eye protection, and are designed to prevent spread of infection from health care giver to client or from client to health care giver.

Hand Washing

Hand washing is the most important measure in controlling the spread of microorganisms. The Centers for Disease Control (CDC) recommends that health care professionals, such as massage therapists, routinely wash their hands in certain situations. Situations that require routine hand washing include:

Before coming in contact with a client

Between clients (particularly those with high susceptibility to infection)

After caring for an infected client

Before and after handling dressings or touching open wounds

After handling contaminated equipment (e.g., sheets, towels)

Body Substance Isolation (BSI)

BSI is a set of guidelines that provides a consistent approach to managing body substances from all patients and is essential to prevent spread of infection. The infection precautions used in BSI place a physical barrier between the caregiver and potentially infectious agents. Consistent barrier precautions should be used whenever there is a chance of coming into contact with a client's broken skin or moist body substances (e.g., blood, pus, feces, urine, saliva). Some of the precautionary measures recommended for massage therapists in clinic and hospital settings include gloves, gowns, masks, and proper hygiene.

Gloves

Gloves should be changed between patient contacts, but are not necessary for contact with unsoiled articles or intact skin. Wearing gloves should not be a substitute for hand washing.

Gowns

Gowns are worn to provide a barrier between the clothing and body of both the client and care giver. Gowns are also used to protect against splashing of body substances.

Masks

Masks provide a barrier to airborne diseases.

Hygiene

Hygiene and proper cleanliness are absolutely essential elements in massage therapy. All bodyworkers and clients should be taught to practice proper hygiene, such as frequent body and hand washing, especially when dealing with infection.

For the therapist, **overall hygiene** includes:

Bathing daily
Keeping nails trimmed and clean
Keeping clothes clean with unscented detergents
Avoiding colognes and perfumes (clients may have aversions or sensitivities to certain scents)
Keeping fresh breath and avoiding breathing directly on the client

Therapists should also be diligent about cleanliness of the **hands and arms:**

Wash your hands before and after each massage.
Be sure to use an antibacterial soap and wash thoroughly with hot water.
In the clinic setting, use single-use towels.

Contraindications and Indications for Common Disorders

Following is an alphabetized list of the contraindications and indications for some of the most common disorders seen in a clinical setting. Because most of these disorders and conditions are described in detail in the CLINICAL PATHOLOGY section, only a brief description of each condition is given here. The main intent of the remainder of this chapter is to provide a quick reference list for the contraindications and indications of massage for some of the more common disorders and conditions. Refer to the individual chapters in the CLINICAL PATHOLOGY section for information regarding signs, symptoms, and causes for any of these disorders.

Abdominal aneurysm — localized abnormal dilation of a blood vessel, usually an artery, resulting in the vessel wall becoming weak and distorted; dangerous if it ruptures.
Contraindications/Indications: massage of abdomen is contraindicated.

Abnormal lumps — tissue growth inconsistent with normal tissue.
Contraindications/Indications: avoid the immediate area and diplomatically suggest the client see a doctor.

Abnormal sensations — sensations that may occur as a symptom of certain conditions (e.g., diabetes, stroke, hyperesthesia, neurologic disorders) or as a side effect of some medications; can signal a problem.
Contraindications/Indications: be cautious; research the condition; obtain doctor's approval, if necessary.

Acne — inflammation of the sebaceous glands and hair *follicles.*
Contraindications/Indications: not contagious; avoid massage if affected areas are painful, itching, or weeping.

Alzheimer's disease — a chronic, organic mental disorder; a form of presenile dementia due to atrophy of the frontal and occipital lobes of the brain; includes irreversible loss of intellectual functions; onset is usually between 40 and 60 years of age.
Contraindications/Indications: massage may sooth muscular spasm, improve motor function, and improve psychologic well-being; consult client's doctor before

beginning therapy; strongly consider having a family member or friend accompany the client during massage sessions.

Amputation — to cut off a projecting part (e.g., limb, breast).

  Contraindications/Indications: use caution around broken skin; tapotement and other tissue manipulation can increase circulation and reduce scar tissue.

Amyotrophic lateral sclerosis (Lou Gehrig's disease) — a syndrome marked by muscular weakness and atrophy with palsy; caused by degeneration of motor neurons of the spinal cord, medulla, and cortex.

  Contraindications/Indications: massage may sooth muscular spasm and improve motor function and psychologic well-being; may need to consult client's doctor.

Anemia — a condition in which there is reduced delivery of oxygen to the tissues due to increased destruction or decreased production of erythrocytes (red blood cells).

  Contraindications/Indications: extreme fluid movement or pressure on surface vessels may be harmful; massage should be light and soothing.

Angina pectoris — pain in the chest due to reduced coronary circulation that may or may not be due to heart or arterial disorders, myocardial infarction, hypertensive heart disease, or any of the chronic ischemic heart diseases.

  Contraindications/Indications: all massage should be light and soothing; avoid endangerment areas and abdominal massage (may cause increased pressure on the heart); client is best positioned supine with a cushion under the right hip to avoid pressure on the inferior vena cava; massage can overwork the heart, so check with client's doctor before performing any bodywork.

Arteriosclerosis — a number of pathologic conditions in which there is thickening and hardening of the arteries.

  Contraindications/Indications: avoid localized massage around the carotid artery (may break loose plaque); no deep tissue work; get doctor's approval before starting therapy.

Arthritis — includes rheumatoid arthritis and osteoarthritis.

  Rheumatoid arthritis — a chronic, systemic disease that causes inflammatory changes and results in crippling deformities.

    Contraindications/Indications: avoid affected joints when in an acute and inflamed stage; paraffin bath is the medical treatment of choice.

  Osteoarthritis — a chronic disease characterized by degeneration of articular cartilage, spurs, and bone growths; usually occurs in weight-bearing joints.

    Contraindications/Indications: very slow range of movement is indicated; avoid friction of affected areas. If the spine is affected (**degenerative disk disease**): check with client's doctor before starting therapy; possibly avoid affected area during acute phase; massage can prevent contracture or inhibit associated protection of the affected disk.

Asthma — a condition characterized by constriction of the bronchial airways; sometimes related to stress.

  Contraindications/Indications: massage can reduce stress and loosen the intercostal muscles; any bodywork should be relaxing; deep work can cause stress or pain, which can trigger an episode.

Atherosclerosis — the most common form of arteriosclerosis; deposits of plaque made up of fats and cholesterol form in the arteries, causing them to harden and thicken; eventually alters the function of the tissues.

  Contraindications/Indications: avoid areas of concern (i.e., posterior tibial, popliteal, femoral, axillary, brachial, radial, carotid, and temporal arteries); general massage is contraindicated in severe cases because fluid movement could cause an embolism (i.e., blood vessel clogged by a foreign substance or blood clot).

Bell's palsy — unilateral facial paralysis presumed to be caused by swelling of the seventh cranial nerve (i.e., the facial nerve) at the cervical spine.